Bone Management in Dental Implantology

Andi Setiawan Budihardja • Thomas Mücke
Editors

Bone Management in Dental Implantology

Springer

Editors
Andi Setiawan Budihardja
Oral and Maxillofacial Surgery
University of Pelita Harapan Jakarta
Tangerang
Indonesia

Department of Oral Maxillofacial Surgery
Faculty of Medicine, Siloam Hospital
Lippo Village
University Pelita Harapan
Tangerang
Banten
Indonesia

Budihardja Dental Specialist Center
Jakarta
Indonesia

Thomas Mücke
Head of the Department of Oral and
Maxillofacial and Plastic Surgery
Malteser Clinic Krefeld-Uerdingen
North Rhine-Westfalia
Germany

Technische Universität München,
Klinikum rechts der Isar
München
Germany

ISBN 978-3-319-78950-7 ISBN 978-3-319-78951-4 (eBook)
https://doi.org/10.1007/978-3-319-78951-4

This Springer imprint is published by the registered company Springer Nature Switzerland AG
The registered company address is: Gewerbestrasse 11, 6330 Cham, Switzerland

Foreword

Implantology represents a fascinating part of dentistry. Although most situations can be solved without major additional surgical procedures and the insertion of implants can thus be performed successfully, there are an increasing number of patients with atrophic or otherwise unsuitable jaws. Without bone there is no way to insert implants. Therefore, bone augmentation is an essential part of the armamentarium to overcome these atrophic anatomical situations and increase the availability of implants to the benefit of our patients.

Bone augmentation starts with simple bone grafts and ranges to the most complex bone augmentation with microsurgical composite bone flaps. Advanced techniques in GBR can be used to repair severe horizontal and vertical bone defects. Various biomaterials can be used to enhance bone formation; however autogenous bone is still the gold standard in dental implantology.

This book describes all the reader needs to know about bone augmentation in dental implantology. Advantages and disadvantages such as patient donor site morbidities are discussed. The key messages of this book are guided by both scientific knowledge and personal experience. Surgical procedures are illustrated with many case examples in colorful detail. This book is of great benefit for anybody interested in bone augmentation techniques to improve and widen the scope of their dental implantology.

Frank Hölzle, MD, DMD, PhD, FEBOMFS
Chairman Klinik für Mund
Kiefer und Gesichtschirurgie
Uniklinik RWTH Aachen
Aachen
Germany

Preface

Writing a book is mandatory in academics for their students and colleagues. This is important to develop knowledge and exchange experience in a particular field of specialization.

The field of dental implantology in the past few years has expanded rapidly. Insertion of dental implant nowadays has been done not only to a patient with a good bone condition but also to those with severe bone defects. This has its own challenges to a clinician.

In the past few decades, many techniques and materials have been developed to be able to reconstruct bone defects. Even though there are a lot of controversions, the use of autogenous bone is still a gold standard in dental implantology. The application of an autogenous bone can be done in a form of pure autogenous bone or a combination of autogenous bone and guided bone regeneration (GBR) to decrease patient morbidity.

Expansion of rapid biomaterial, although have not replaced autogenous bone, cannot be denied have managed the operator to do a complex bone augmentation in a simpler way and less invasive. Complex bone augmentation procedures nowadays can be learned and applied easily by the clinicians. It can be applied with more predictable results with less complication.

This book discusses various techniques of bone augmentation in dental implantology, which according to the writer can be applied in daily practice.

Distinguished colleagues have contributed to the writing of several chapters relevant to their field of specialization. We would like to thank all the authors and contributors for their valuable contribution.

We would like also to express our gratitude to our teachers and role models in this field:

- Prof.Dr.Dr. K.-D.Wolff. Chairman Klinik für Mund, Kiefer und Gesichtschirurgie, Klinikum rechts der Isar, Technische Universität, München, Germany
- Prof.Dr.Dr. Frank. Hölzle. Chairman Klinik für Mund, Kiefer und Gesichtschirurgie, Uniklinik RWTH Aachen, Germany
- Dr.Dr. Christoph Pytlik, Germany
- Dr. Masykur Rahmat (+), Yogyakarta, Indonesia

Last but not least, we would like to thank our family, Dr. Juwana Budihardja (+), Dr. Katrin Liwoto, Devi, Keisha, Nathan, Debby, and Anita, for their patient, continuous support throughout the entire process of writing this book.

Tangerang, Indonesia — Andi Setiawan Budihardja
North Rhine-Westfalia, Germany — Thomas Mücke

Contents

Basic Principle in Bone Augmentation

1

Andi Setiawan Budihardja and Mimi Kallmann

1.1 Introduction

The most important determinant of success of treatment with dental implants is the availability of adequate bone structure. In order for dental implants to be successful, the bone must be both sufficient quantitatively (with regard to height and/or width) and qualitatively (ample vascularization) (Figs. 1.1 and 1.2).

A lack of adequate bone structure is a common deterrent to placing dental implants and also a common cause of failed implants after placement, both in the healing/osseointegration phase and in the restoration phase.

There are several circumstances that can lead to loss of bone, namely:

- Genetic defects (i.e., cleft lip/palate) (Fig. 1.3).
- Trauma.
- Tumor and postablative tumor surgery (Fig. 1.4).
- Bone atrophy.
- Infection.
- Periodontal disease.

A. S. Budihardja (✉)
Department of Oral and Maxillofacial Surgery, Faculty of Medicine, University Pelita Harapan, Jakarta, Indonesia

Siloam Hospital Lippo Village, Jakarta, Indonesia

Budihardja Dental Specialist Center, Jakarta, Indonesia

M. Kallmann
Private Practice, Jakarta, Indonesia

A. S. Budihardja, T. Mücke (eds.), *Bone Management in Dental Implantology*,
https://doi.org/10.1007/978-3-319-78951-4_1

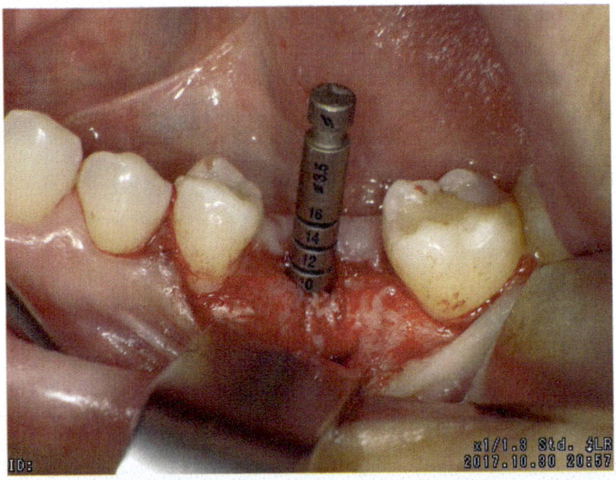

Fig. 1.1 Dental implant must be covered by a healthy bone and soft tissue. It should be placed in the correct 3-D position

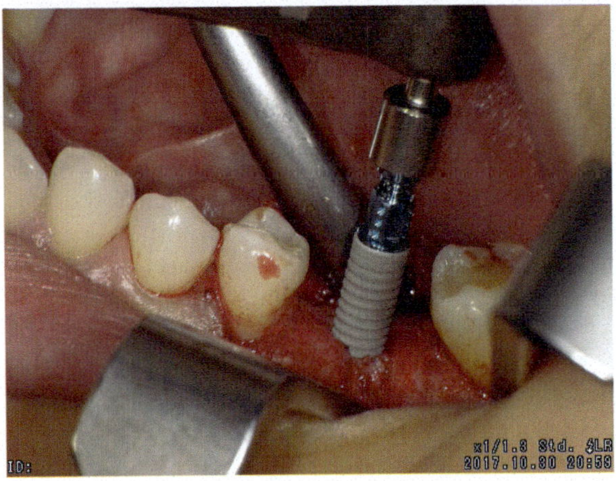

Fig. 1.2 Dental implant insertion on healthy bone

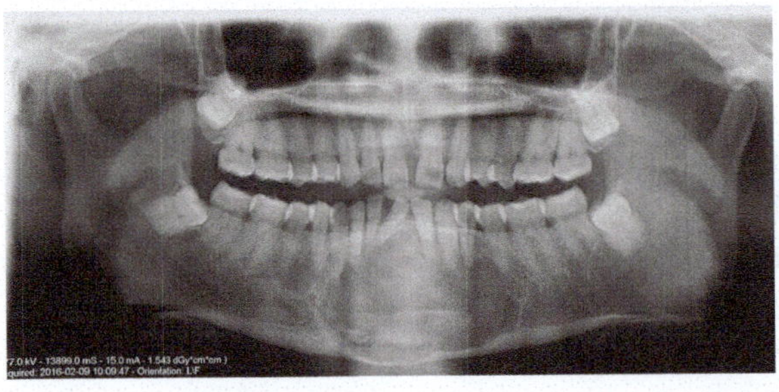

Fig. 1.3 Ameloblastoma (benign tumor) of the anterior mandible resulting in severe bone destruction

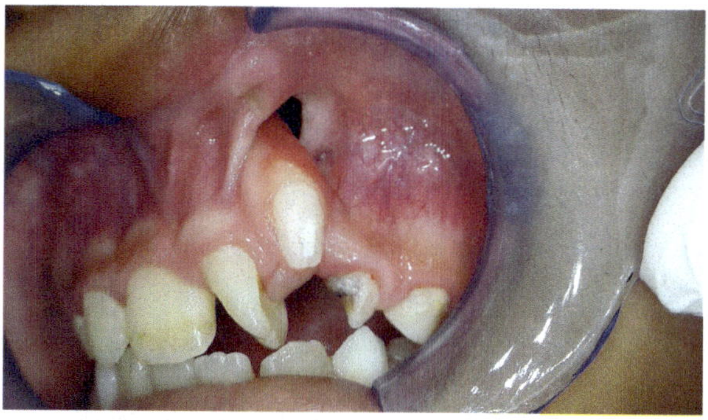

Fig. 1.4 Alveolar bone defect on the patient with unilateral cleft lip and palate

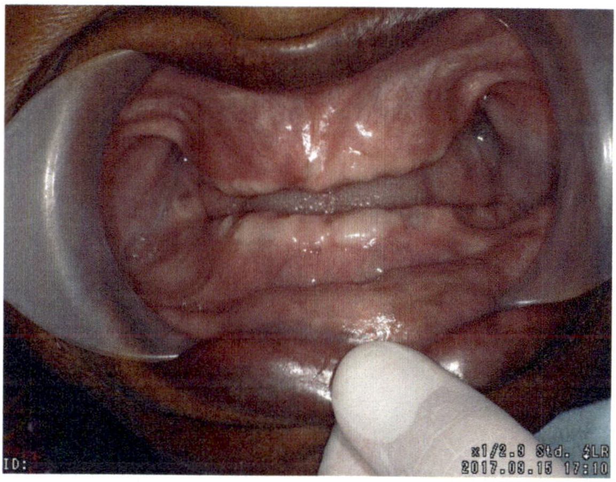

Fig. 1.5 Resorption of the upper jaw in the centripetal direction and the lower jaw in a centrifugal pattern. This will lead to a pseudo-class III occlusion

1.2 Bone Quantity

Tooth loss means a loss of functional loading, which can lead to resorption and atrophy of the jaw. This situation can be further aggravated if the teeth are not replaced for a substantial time, if the patient uses dentures, and if there is any inflammation or infection after tooth extraction. Bone resorption begins at week 15 post tooth extraction and reaches approximately 60% within a period of 3 years (Fig. 1.5). Resorption of the mandible is fourfold faster than in the maxilla. Mandibular resorption occurs around 12 mm in the first year after extraction, from which point it increases by about 0.2 mm per year [1, 2]. Maxillary resorption is in a centripetal direction, whereas mandibular resorption has a centrifugal pattern (Figs. 1.4 and 1.6) [3]. For this reason, there are often discrepancies in the relationship between the upper and lower jaw. This can result in pseudo-class III malocclusion jaw relationship.

Changes in bone structure would also result in changes to soft tissue structure and ultimately would have an impact on the patient's profile. This is all too common a cause of aesthetic problems in patients.

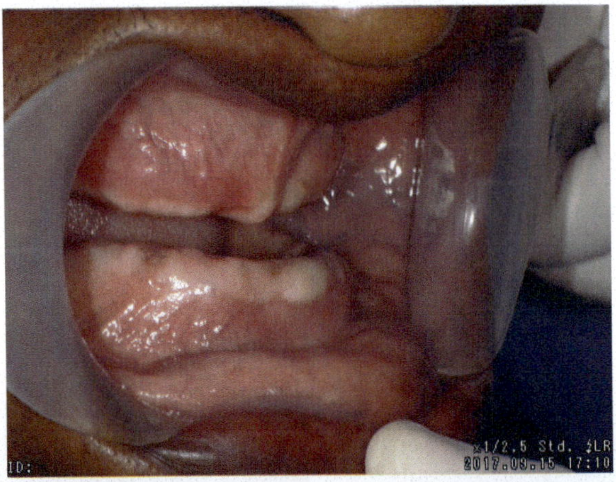

Fig. 1.6 Resorption of the upper jaw in the centripetal direction and the lower jaw in a centrifugal pattern. This will lead to a pseudo-class III occlusion

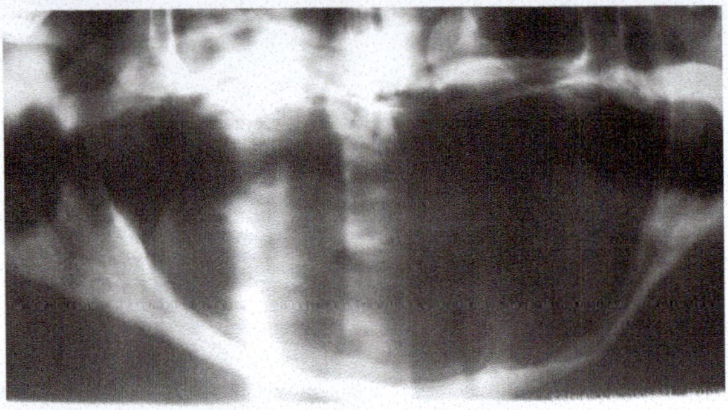

Fig. 1.7 Edentulous jaw with severe bone resorption. In such circumstances, the danger of mandibular fracture is considerable

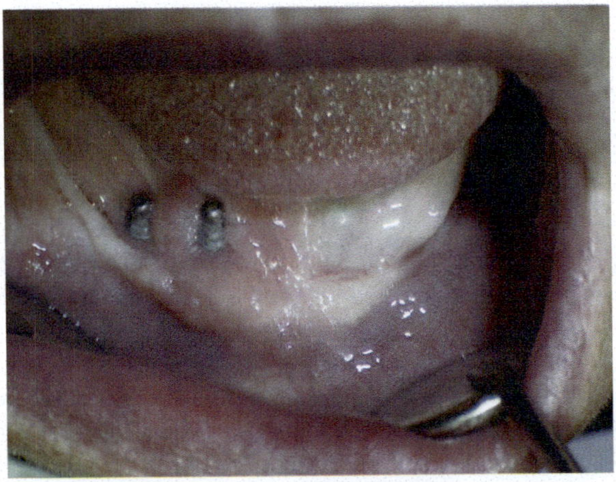

Fig. 1.8 Insertion of four implants in interforaminal region in severely atrophic jaw. Inclination of the implants is too far to the lingual side because it was forced to match the prosthetic on the upper jaw. This patient has a pseudo-class III occlusion because of the jaw resorption on the edentulous upper and lower jaw. It is well described in the literature that such case can cause life-threatening complication because of the hematoma from the floor of the mouth and bleeding that can cause obstruction of the airway

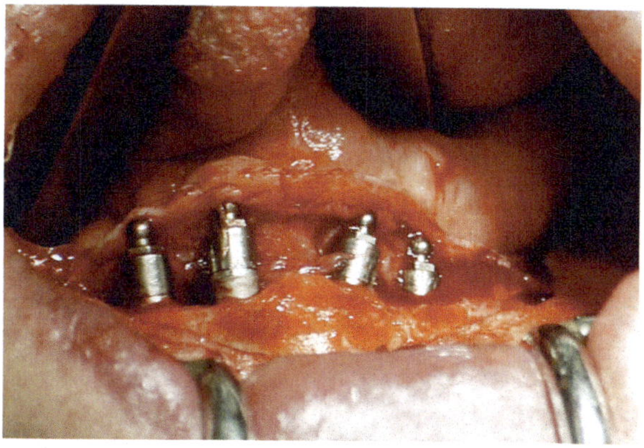

Fig. 1.9 Insertion of four implants in interforaminal region in severely atrophic jaw. Inclination of the implants is too far to the lingual side because it was forced to match the prosthetic on the upper jaw. This patient has a pseudo-class occlusion because of the jaw resorption on the edentulous upper and lower jaw. It is well described in the literature that such case can cause life-threatening complication because of the hematoma from the floor of the mouth and bleeding that can cause obstruction of the airway

Tooth loss, if not corrected in a timely fashion, not only causes changes in the hard tissue (bone) but also can lead to changes in the soft tissues, including the muscles of the face (Figs. 1.7, 1.8, and 1.9).

1.3 Bone Quality

Bone quality is a major prognostic factor for the success of dental implants. Bone vitality is determined by bone vascularity and intraosseous cellular components of the bone. Some comorbidities may cause interference with bone vitality, such as diabetes mellitus, osteoporosis, and other bone diseases (osteomalacia, postradiation malignancies, etc. (Fig. 1.10)).

The use of bisphosphonate drugs, whether administered intravenously or orally, has an inhibitory effect on osteoclasts, resulting in poor vitality. Patients treated with bisphosphonate therapy often have resultant osteonecrosis of the jaw after undergoing dental surgery (Figs. 1.11, 1.12, 1.13, and 1.14); there have even been several cases of osteonecrosis which occurs spontaneously, without prior surgery of any kind (e.g., due to prosthesis pressure or in cases of chronic periodontitis). However, patient under bisphosphonate therapy is not absolute contraindication for dental implant surgery and bone grafting. Several publications reported dental implant surgery and bone grafting could be done successfully in patient under low-dose oral bisphosphonate therapy [4, 5].

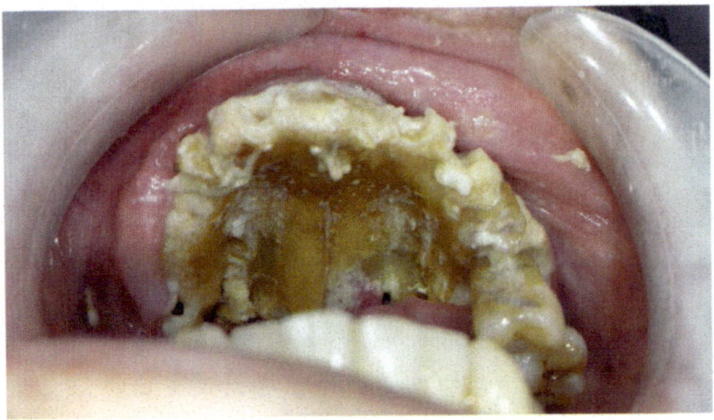

Fig. 1.10 Osteomyelitis of the maxilla post radiotherapy

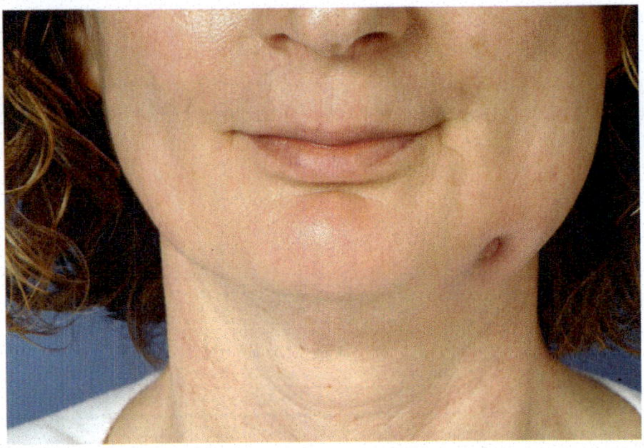

Fig. 1.11 Patient with bisphosphonate-related osteonecrosis of the jaw. Osteonecrosis of the mandible occurs after tooth extraction. Patient received i.v. bisphosphonate therapy after breast carcinoma operation

Determination of these bony structures can only be made clinically and histologically. The use of CT scans (based on Hounsfield scale) can determine the degree of bone mineralization, but cannot measure the vitality and precisely discern the bone structure. This can only be accurately accomplished by histological examination. For this reason, using radiographic examinations to predict prognosis is considered inaccurate.

1.4 Principle of Bone Grafting

The main principle of bone grafting is to attempt to avoid having to do a bone graft. In other words, try to find a viable alternative before deciding to do a bone graft. Alternatives to this procedure are imperative, because although there are several techniques of bone grafting that have promising prognoses, bone grafting is nevertheless an invasive surgical procedure and as such carries risk of complications. In addition, bone grafting will incur considerable additional costs for the patient. Several strategies for avoiding the need for a bone graft are as follows:

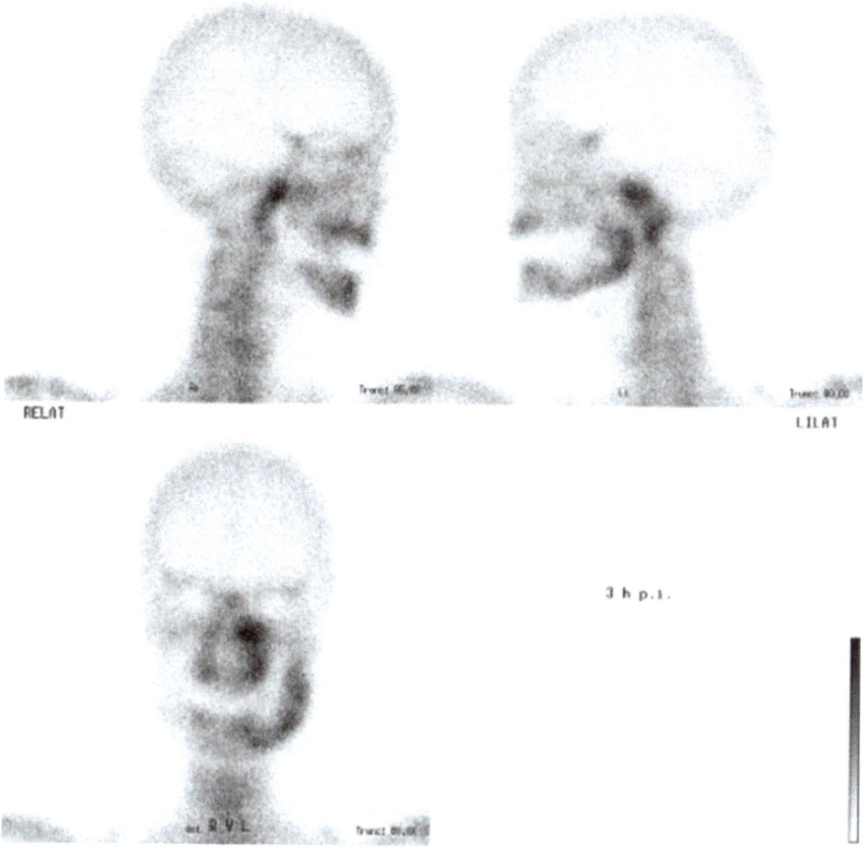

Fig. 1.12 Bone scintigraphy shows an area of osteonecrosis of the left mandible

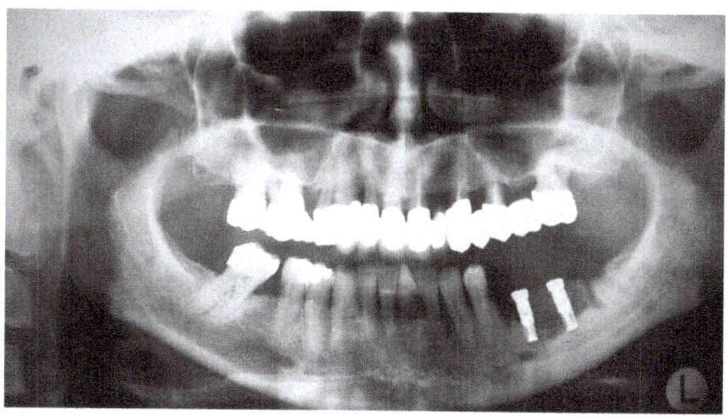

Fig. 1.13 Dental implants on the mandible were inserted in the patient with the history of taking i.v. bisphosphonate therapy for breast cancer. Implants failed to osseointegrate and have to be removed. Moreover, all necrotic bones have to be removed and local flaps are needed to close soft tissue defect

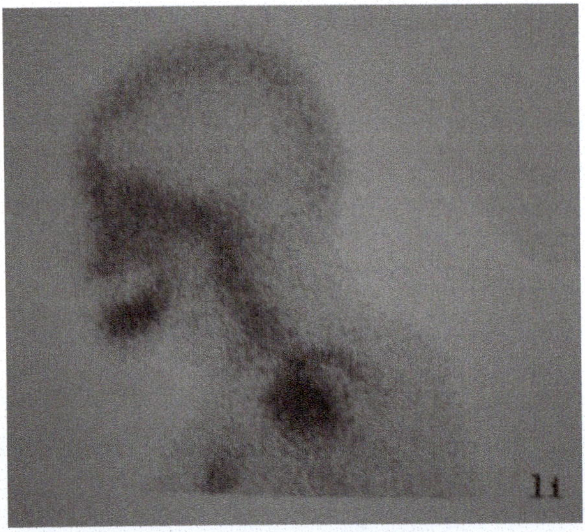

Fig. 1.14 Bone scintigraphy shows a necrotic bone on the mandible

1.4.1 Implantation Immediately After Extraction/Immediate Implant Placement

Placement of dental implants performed immediately after extraction or performed 4–6 weeks after extraction (after allowing time for soft tissue healing) can prevent bone resorption, thus avoiding the need for a bone graft at a later date. Immediate implant placement is considered as a complex surgical procedure. It requires high surgical skill to place implant in a correct 3-D position and to get primary stability. Soft tissue recession is one of the major disadvantages of immediate implant placement. This can be caused by malpositioned implant placement and also by facial bone resorption. Immediate implant placement can be used in ideal conditions with thick bone wall, thick soft tissue phenotypes, and where dental implant can be inserted in correct 3-D position with primary stability. Failure to place implant in correct 3-D position is a major factor that leads to periimplantitis.

1.5 Timing of Implant Placement [6]

Type	Description
1	Immediate implant placement
2	Early implant placement with soft tissue healing (4–6 weeks)
3	Early implant placement with partial bone healing (12–16 weeks)
4	Late implant placement in healed sites (6 months or more)

An advantage of placing dental implants 4–6 weeks after tooth extraction, compared with immediate placement (on the same day as extraction), is that it allows for

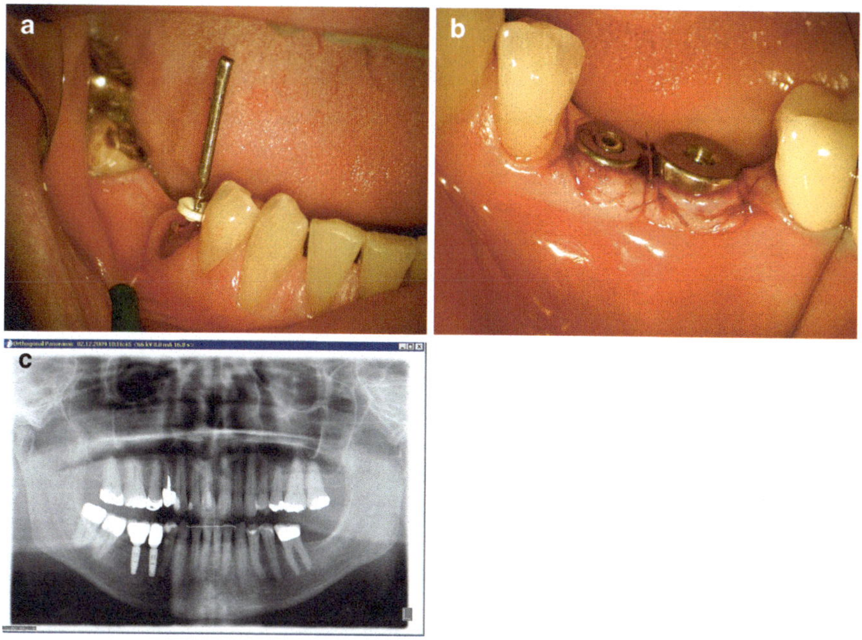

Fig. 1.15 (a–c) Atraumatic extraction of tooth 44 followed by immediate implant placement on tooth 44. Orthopantomogram after prosthetic restoration showed good osseointegration with stable bone formation around dental implants

primary healing of the soft tissues, reducing the need for extensive periosteal releasing incision or soft tissue graft to achieve primary closure of the soft tissue (Fig. 1.15a–c). It also allows to place dental implant in correct 3-D position. Early implant placement also allows acute or chronic infection to heal completely.

After 4 months the prosthetic part can be corrected to adapt new soft tissue condition after healing period (Figs. 1.16 and 1.17).

Multi-rooted teeth are relative contraindication for immediate implant placement. Immediate implant placement in teeth with multiple roots often leads to complications. Placement in the central part of the septum often results in instability and failure to achieve osseointegration. Placement in one of the extraction sockets will result in an imbalance in the prosthodontic restoration. The placement of two implants in two sockets will result in poor prosthodontic restoration that is not consistent with the anatomical crown shape.

1.5.1 Placement of Dental Implants in Interforaminal and Intermaxillary Sinus

Placement of dental implants in the interforaminal mandibular area and intermaxillary sinus of the maxillary area can avoid the need for bone grafting and/or sinus augmentation surgery. Prosthodontic restoration can be accomplished through the utilization

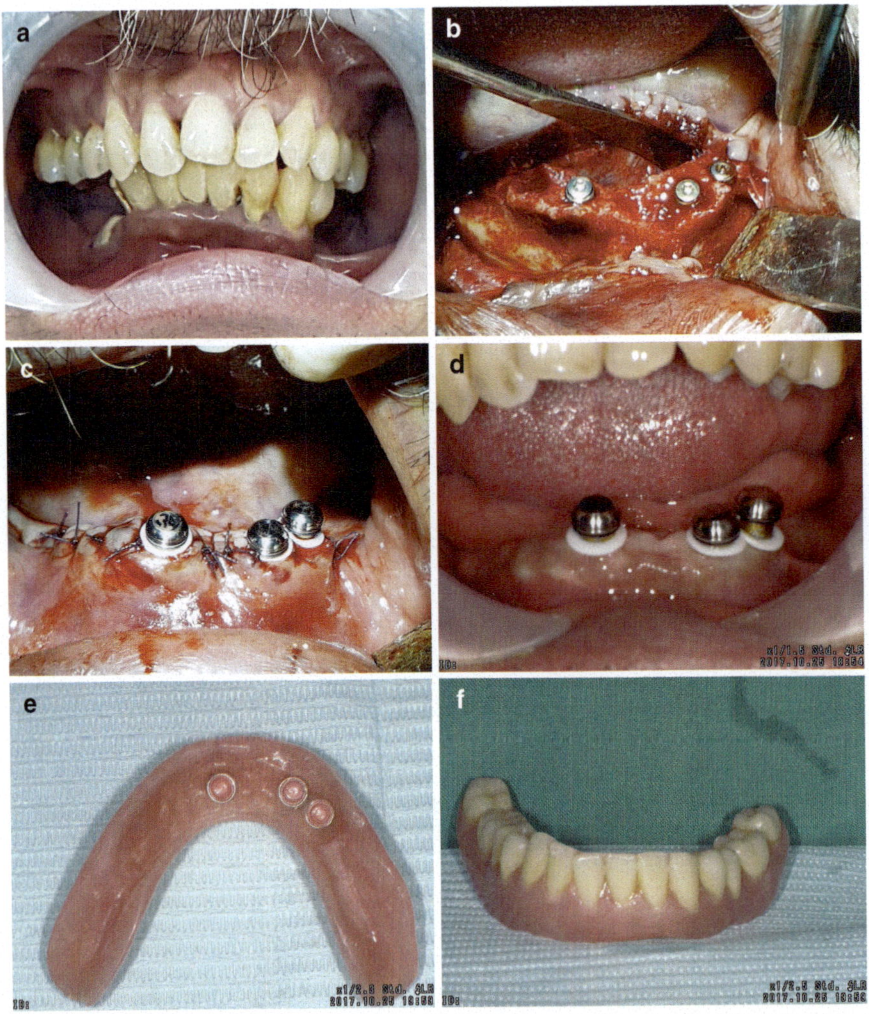

Fig. 1.16 (**a–f**) Immediate implant insertion after extraction of hopeless teeth in the anterior mandible. Prosthetic restoration using hybrid denture can be done at the same day. This will reduce treatment time, prevent the need of major bone grafting, and increase patient comfort

of removable dentures, bonded to the implant using either bar, magnet, conical, or telescopic attachments (Fig. 1.18a–c, 1.19a, b, and 1.20a, b). The benefits are minimal surgery, a relatively inexpensive price, and results in stable restorations. Additionally, patients can maintain better oral hygiene, because the dentures can be removed and easily cleaned. To achieve good stability, a minimum of four implants were required in the maxilla and minimum of two implants in the mandible. Some dental implant systems allow for immediate loading that can reduce treatment time.

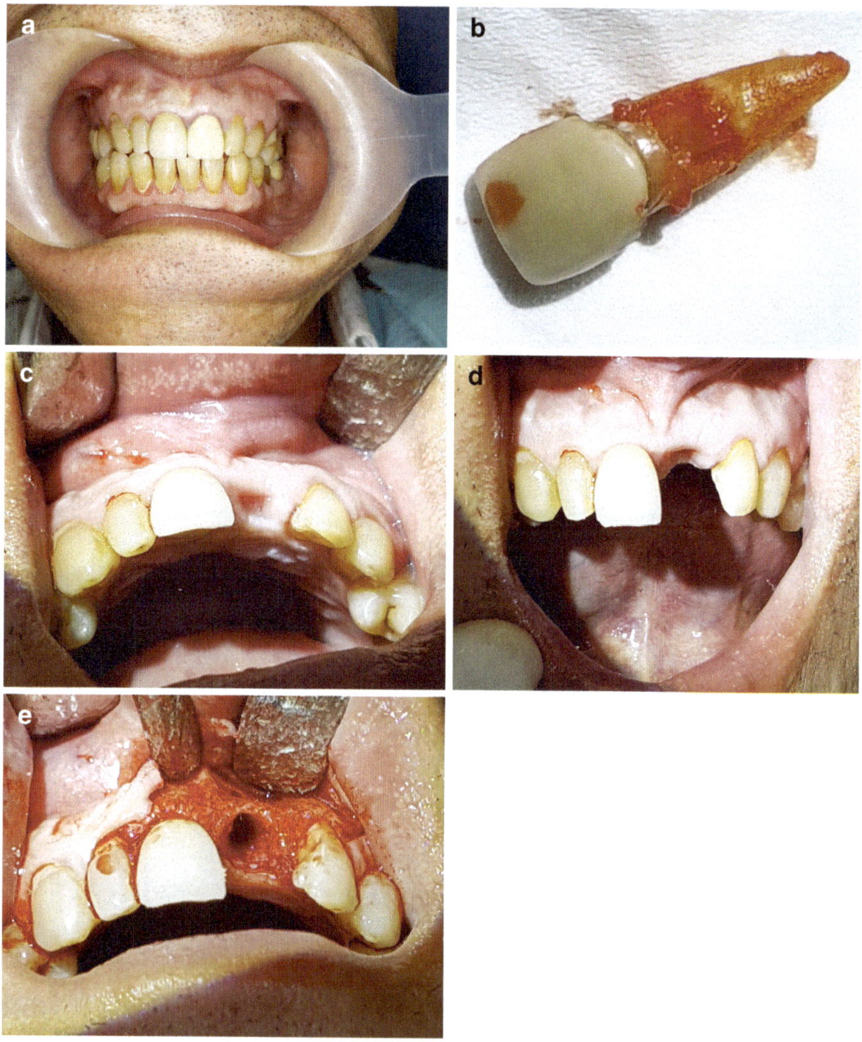

Fig. 1.17 (**a**–**e**) Wound healing after 12 weeks corresponding to type 3 timing for implant insertion. Tooth 21 with severe root resorption that cannot be treated with conventional endodontic treatment was extracted. Dental implant was inserted 12 weeks after tooth extraction in correct 3-D position; soft tissue can be sutured easily without tension and without the need to do extensive periosteal releasing incision even when guided bone regeneration was done simultaneously

1.5.2 The Use of Short Implants (<8 mm) and Mini Implant

Dental implants with a length <8 mm are often propagated for their ability to be used in cases of severe bone resorption. The use of these shorter dental implants is advantageous because bone grafting can be avoided. Deporter et al. [7] reported results of their research using short dental implants, revealing a 10-year implant

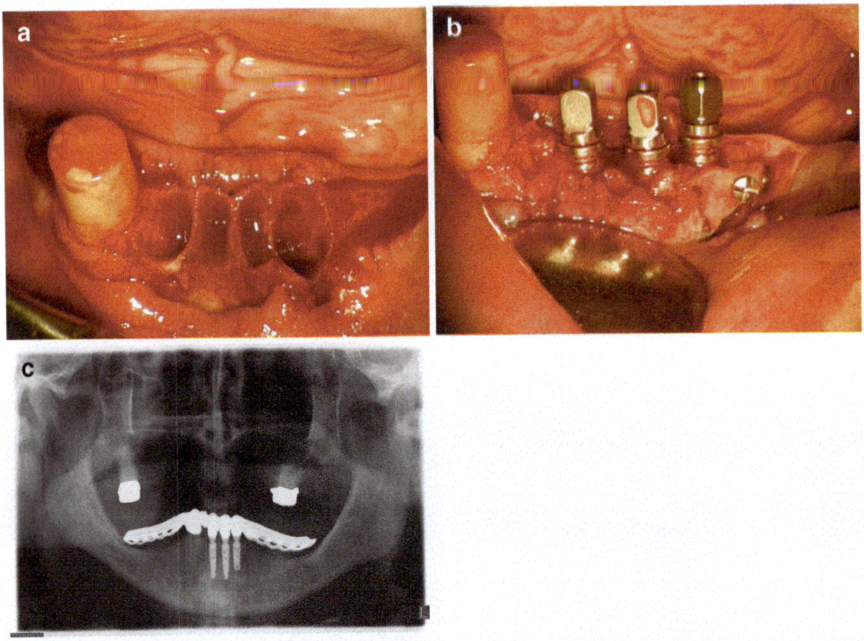

Fig. 1.18 (a–c) Immediate implant placement in the anterior mandible after extraction of hopeless teeth. Hybrid denture attached to the implant. This prosthetic solution can avoid the need of complex bone augmentation

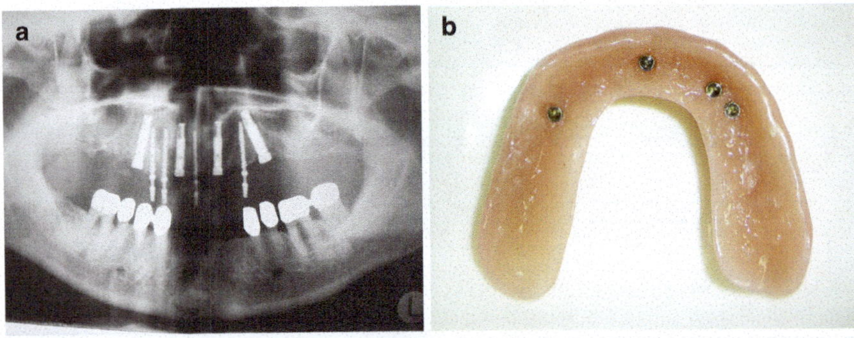

Fig. 1.19 (a, b) Insertion of four dental implants in the intersinus maxillary area. Definitive prosthetic rehabilitation was achieved using hybrid denture. This allows the patient to get optimal result (in terms of denture stability and easiness to maintain good oral hygiene) without major bone augmentation. Directly after implant placement, the patient can wear removable denture that attached to the temporary implants

survival of 92.7%, with an average annual bone loss after 1 year of 0.03 mm. Reviewing the literature the overall survival rate for short implants is over 95% in some studies [8, 9].

Nonetheless, the use of short dental implants has drawbacks as well. Often there is a discrepancy between the implant length and the tooth crown. This has a negative

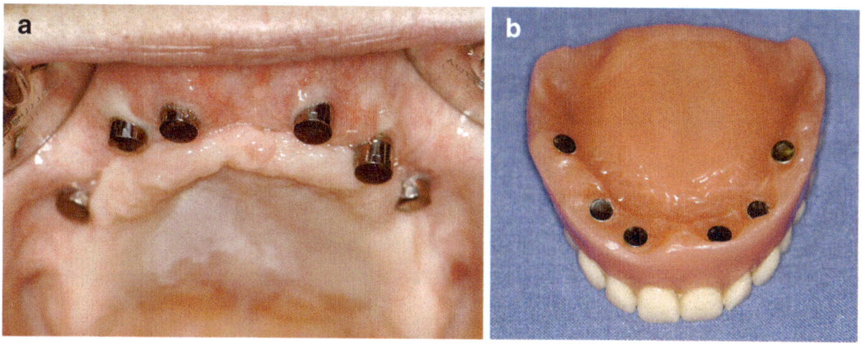

Fig. 1.20 (**a**, **b**) Insertion of six dental implants in the maxilla can avoid the need of complex bone augmentation. Prosthetic rehabilitation was hybrid denture that attached to six dental implants

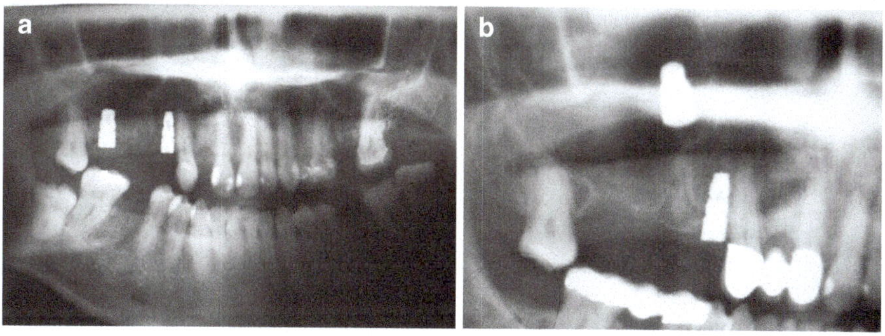

Fig. 1.21 (**a**, **b**) Short dental implant was inserted in a soft bone in the posterior maxilla without a proper bone augmentation procedure. This leads to the loss and migration of implant to the maxillary sinus 2 years after prosthetic rehabilitation

effect on the biomechanical aspects of mastication and often results in disturbances or failure of osseointegration. In addition, there have been several reports of mandibular fracture, associated with the use of short dental implants in an atrophied jaw. The use of short dental implant in the anterior region where the alveolar bone has suffered severe resorption will result in prosthodontic restoration with elongated teeth and aesthetic imperfections.

Placing short implants in the posterior maxilla also increases the failure rate than placing short implants in the mandible (Fig. 1.21a, b). Poor quality of the bone in the posterior maxilla has mechanical effect on the primary stability in comparison to the dense bone [10].

For these reasons, the use of short dental implants has limited indications (Fig. 1.22a, b).

Although, as mentioned above, there are many ways and techniques to avoid the necessity of bone grafting, often the patient presents with such severe bone resorption that placement of dental implants is not feasible. In these cases, interforaminal placement or other methods described above will not suffice, and it is necessary to proceed with surgical bone grafting before dental implants can be successfully placed.

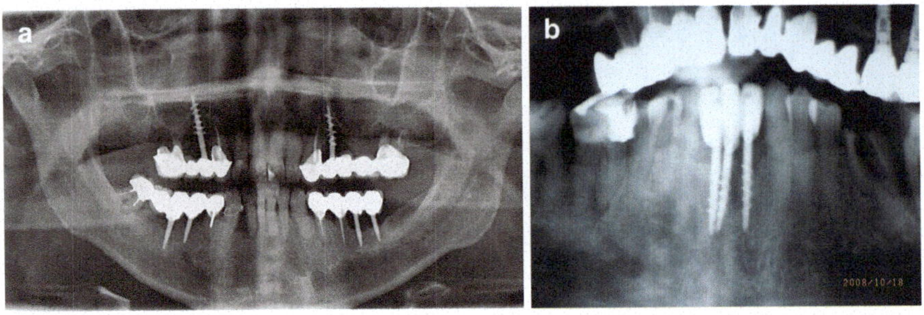

Fig. 1.22 (a, b) A representative case showing mini implants that are used to avoid bone grafting failure because they cannot be placed in the right 3-D position. The prosthetic failure causes failure to the osseointegration

Fig. 1.23 Lateralization of n. alveolaris inferior. This procedure is rarely performed due to the high risk of complications

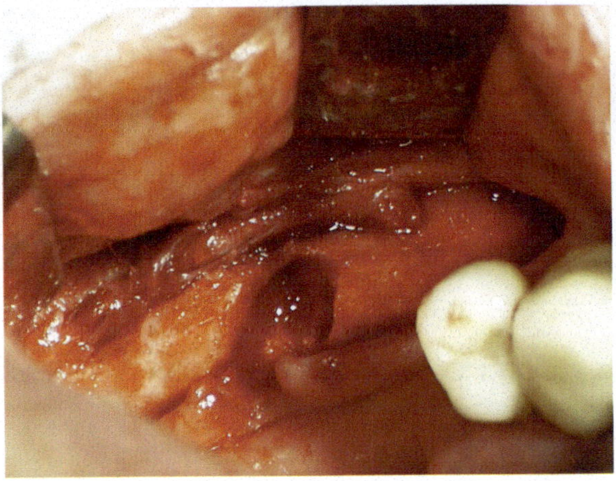

The following methods/procedures can be utilized to manage the bony deficit:

- Bone graft with autogenous bone (for vertical and horizontal bony defects).
- Bone graft with synthetic bone (bone substitute materials, bone tissue engineering).
- Bone graft with a combination of autogenous bone and synthetic bone.
- Distraction osteogenesis.
- Bone splitting (in horizontal bony defects).

The use of distraction osteogenesis is an extremely promising method to handle bony deficits. However, this technique is costly, is time intensive, and is a complex procedure, requiring a highly skilled operator. In-depth discussion on osteogenesis distraction is beyond the scope of this book.

Other techniques, such as nerve lateralization (Fig. 1.23), were previously considered common practice. However, due to the high rate of complications (e.g., paresthesia) even with the most experienced operators, they are no longer considered "state-of-the-art" procedures.

1.6 Classification of Bone Graft Material

Type of material	Origin/source of material
Autograft	Donor and recipient are the same individual There is virtually no risk of graft rejection
Allograft • Fresh-frozen bone allograft • Freeze-dried bone allograft • Demineralized freeze-dried bone allograft • Deproteinized bone allograft	Donor and recipient are genetically distinct, but belong to the same species Risk of graft rejection
Xenograft • Bone material from animal bone • From calcifying corals • From calcifying algae	Donor and recipient have nonidentical genetic composition and belong to different species Risk of graft rejection
Allograft • Calcium phosphate • Carbonate apatite • Bioactive glasses	Biological materials synthesized in a laboratorium Minimal risk of rejection

Autograft is still considered the *gold standard* in dental implantology. This is because this material is the only graft material which has osteogenic, osteoconductive, and osteoinductive properties. In addition, autograft also has mechanical properties (e.g., from cortical bone). Autograft materials are well received by the body, without the risk of rejection or spread of infection/disease.

The downside using autograft material is the donor-site morbidity. Persistent donor-site pain is common for 3–5 days following the harvesting of bone graft. Significant graft resorption is also reported when using autograft. In order to prevent this phenomenon, it is advisable to combine autograft with inorganic bovine bone mineral and collagen membrane. Some modification of the technique also can prevent resorption of autograft.

	Description
Osteogenic	Ability of osteoblasts from the autogenous graft to survive, be nourished by diffusion, and form new vital bone structure
Osteoconductive	Ability of autogenous graft structure to function as “guidance” or a scaffold for vascular proliferation and osteogenesis
Osteoinductive	Ability of bone matrix, mediated by cytokines (BMP, TGF), to induce the process of neoangiogenesis
Biomechanical	Mechanical resistance/strength of cortical bone

1.7 Requirements for Successful Autogenous Bone Graft

- Adequate graft revascularization and close contact and fixation of the graft to the recipient bed.
- Prevent any mechanical stress to the bone grafting area. Providing a good temporary restoration is mandatory in every case.

- Placement of dental implants and removal of osteosynthetic materials are recommended in autogenous bone grafts after a primary healing period of 3–4 months.
- Prolonging the placement of dental implants results in rapid graft resorption; however, removal of osteosynthetics is not recommended before 3 months.
- Using membrane in guided bone regeneration procedure is mandatory to prevent soft tissue ingrowth.

1.8 Autografts Are Further Classified into Vascular and Avascular

1.8.1 Vascular Autogenous Graft

- The bone graft is harvested with blood vessels (arteries and veins) which are then anastomosed using microsurgery technique to the recipient area vasculature (most commonly in the vessels of the neck). The advantages of this method are rapid graft incorporation and minimal cell death, due to the direct supply of nutrients in the blood. The bone and soft tissue can be harvested at the same time when using this graft.
- The disadvantages include requiring a more complex surgery, skilled operator, and considerably high cost for the procedure. In general, this type of grafting is reserved for large reconstructions of the upper and/or lower jaw, posttumor resection, and other malignancies (Fig. 1.24a–f).
- The most common donor areas are the fibula and iliac bone.

1.8.2 Avascular Autograft

1. Intraoral: symphysis, retromolar and edentulous region, and spina nasalis.
2. Extraoral: iliac crest.

Intraoral donor bone can be used for reconstruction of the small and moderate defect. In the past, we were using more bone from the symphysis area, but now we try to avoid donor from the symphysis as much as possible. This is because of the complication that can occur after bone harvesting from this area, such as sensitivity disturbance of the anterior lower teeth and also in the chin area.

For moderate defect intraoral donor from retromolar area can be used. Special instrumentation and technique are needed when harvesting bone from this area.

Extraoral autograft donor can be used for reconstruction of the moderate defect that involved two or more quadrants. A large amount of bone can be harvested from spina iliaca anterior superior (Fig. 1.25a–e). Harvesting bone from anterior is more common in the daily practice, since it does not need to change the position of the patient during the operation. However, several publications have reported that the resorption rate using this graft is higher than intraoral bone. Moreover, the bone consists of more cancellous bone (soft bone). Other extraoral donor sites such as the cranium and tibia are not commonly being use in daily practice.

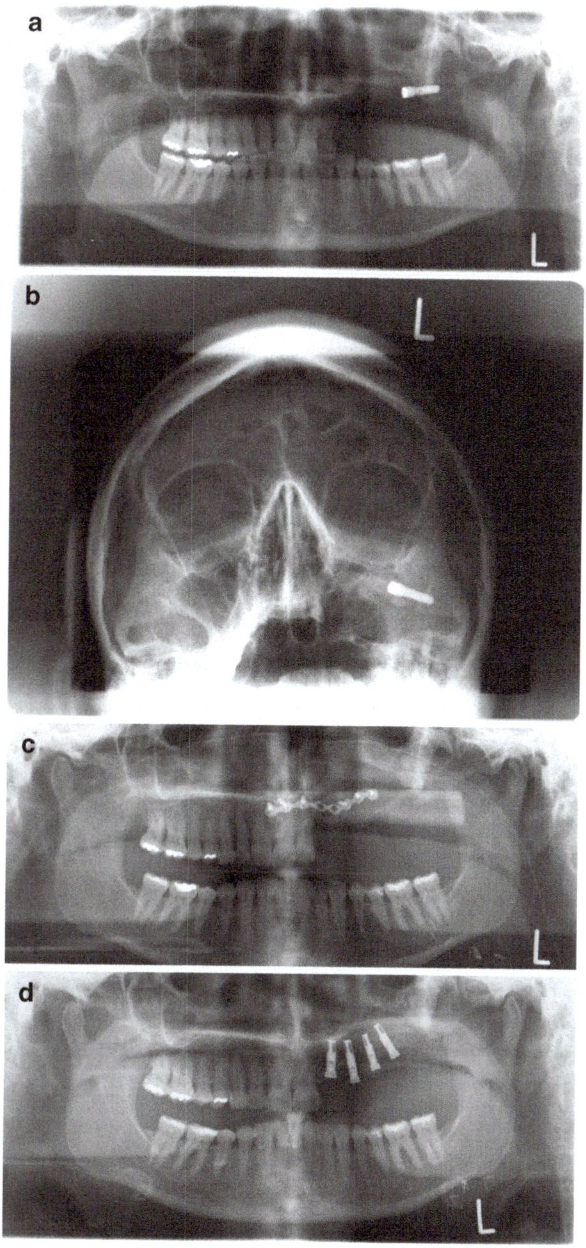

Fig. 1.24 (**a**–**f**) Patient with severe bone defect in the maxilla after hemimaxillectomy surgery to remove malignant tumor in this region. The previous dentist tried to put dental implant in the tuber maxilla area, but this resulted in displacement of the implant because of bone insufficiency. Patient then received a removable obturator denture; however, this denture does not fit patient's satisfaction. The maxilla was then reconstructed using microvascular fibular bone transplant with skin paddle. Four dental implants were inserted in the healed fibula bone. Prosthetic restoration using dental implant was done

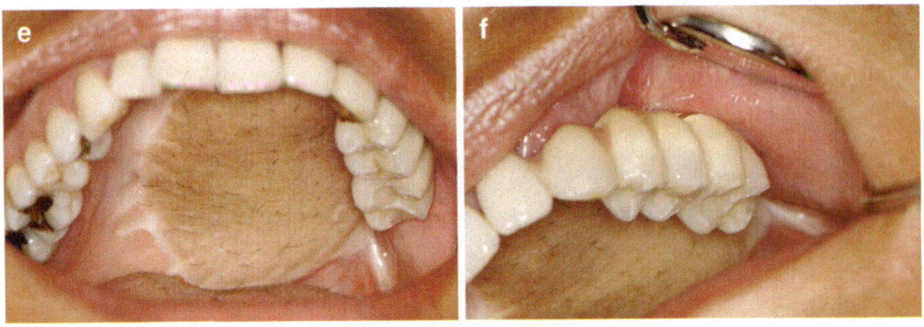

Fig. 1.24 (continued)

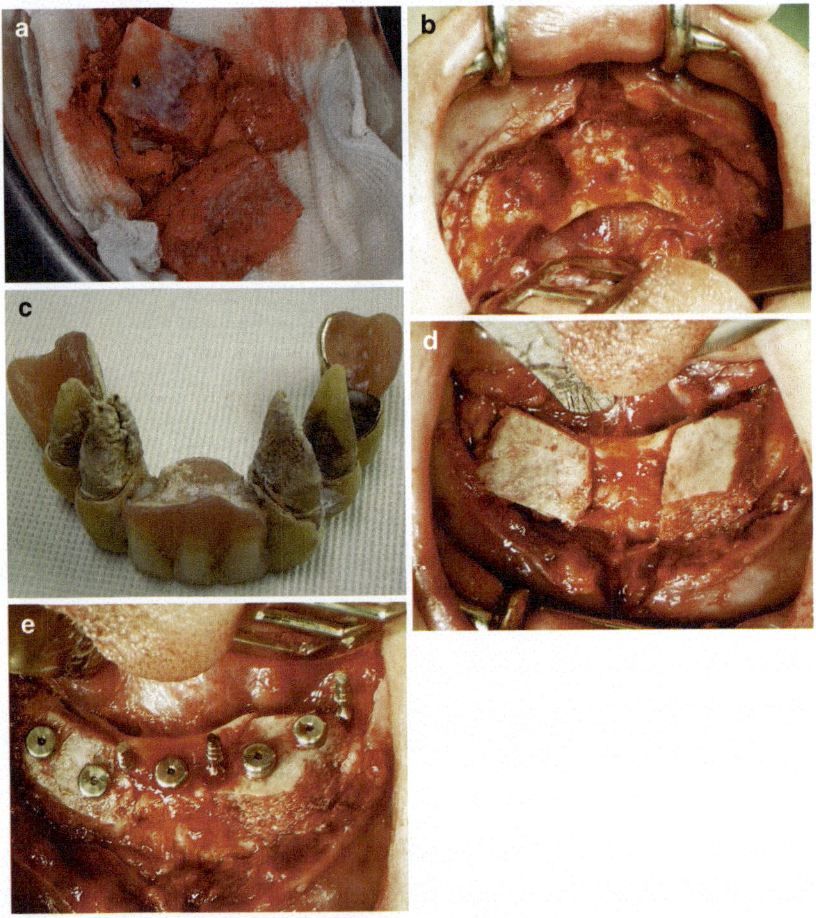

Fig 1.25 (**a–e**) Severe bone defect on the anterior mandible. Patient has removable denture with the teeth that can be removed and then inserted back in the socket by the patient. Bone reconstruction was done with the iliac crest graft. Dental implants were then inserted at the same time. The dental implants have also the function as the "fixation screw" to the block graft. Temporary mini implants were inserted in the original bone for the provisional removable denture to prevent any stress to the grafted bone. Patient could wear the denture directly after operation. Definitive implants were inserted 4 months after bone grafting. Prosthetic restoration was done 3 months after implant insertion. This technique can reduce treatment time and can increase patient comfort

1.9 Membrane

A barrier membrane is used in dental implantology since late 1980. It has been used in the guided bone regeneration procedure to prevent the ingrowth of nonosteogenic connective tissue cells into the regenerating bone defect. Ideal criteria of membrane include biocompatibility, cell occlusion, stability, easy handling, tissue integration, space-making capability, and susceptibility to complication [11–13].

Membranes are classified into resorbable and nonresorbable membranes.

	Advantages	Disadvantages
Nonresorbable membrane • PTFE • ePTFE • ePTFE, titanium reinforced • Titanium	• More stability • Longer barrier function • Can be used for more complex vertical and horizontal augmentation	• Second surgical procedure to remove membrane • Membrane exposure
Resorbable membrane • Synthetic • Allogene • Bovine, porcine, equine	• No need of membrane removal • Easy surgical handling • Faster vascularization	• Membrane collapse • Shorter-duration barrier function • Cannot be used for complex vertical and horizontal augmentation

1.10 Soft Tissue Closure

Soft tissue closure without tension is mandatory when performing any bone augmentation procedure. Failure to do so will result in early dehiscence of the wound. There are two ways to get primary wound closure without tension:

1. Using buccal mucosal flap by doing careful periosteal releasing incision.
2. Using lingual or palatal flap that raised and also carefully do periosteal releasing incision.

Using a good suture material is also important. Generally it is recommended to use monofilament 3.0, 4.0, or 5.0 sutures or PTFE suture material (Fig. 1.26).

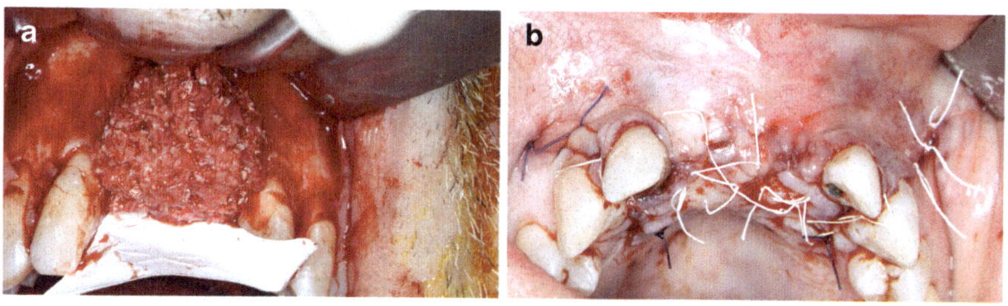

Fig. 1.26 (a–b) Soft tissue closure after bone augmentation procedure in the anterior maxilla. Tension-free mattress suture using a combination of 3.0 and 4.0 PTFE suture was performed

1.11 Temporary Restoration

During healing period, bone graft should be left undisturbed (Figs. 1.27 and 1.28). Stress from the temporary denture to the transplanted bone is one of the factors that can lead to the failure (Figs. 1.29a–c).

The whole treatment with bone graft procedure can take weeks until years period of time. Leaving the patient during this healing procedure without any adequate temporary restoration can lead to the physicosocial problem and often not accepted the patient. Therefore, making a good temporary restoration is an important factor (Figs. 1.27 and 1.28).

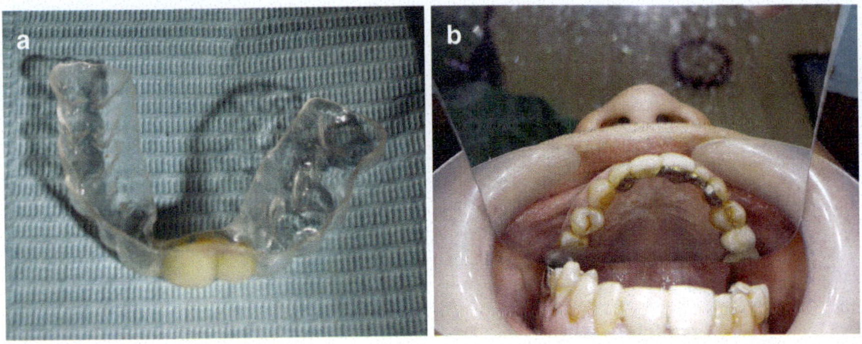

Fig. 1.27 (**a**, **b**) A vacuform retainer (Essix) or rochette bridge can be used as a temporary restoration after grafting procedure

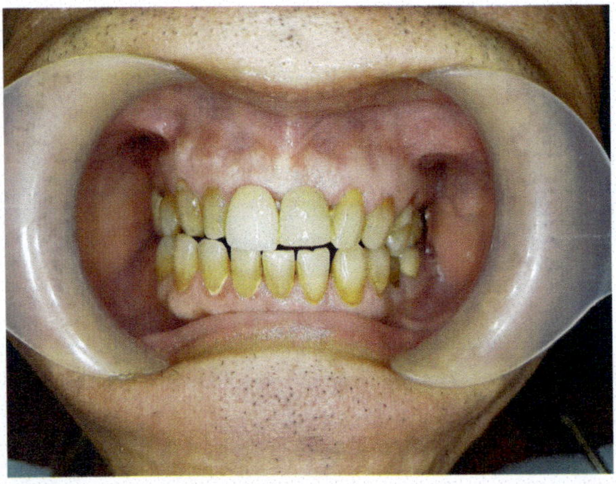

Fig. 1.28 Using Rochette bridge/Maryland bridge as a temporary restoration

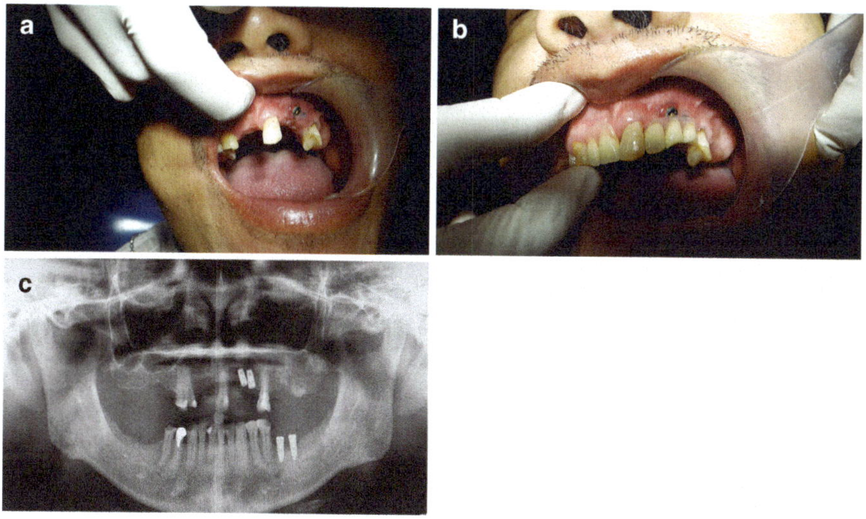

Fig. 1.29 (**a**–**c**) Dental implants that were inserted with simultaneous GBR procedure in the anterior maxilla. These two malpositioned dental implants developed to abscess with purulent pus. Patient was sent home after implantation with removable denture that causes constant pressure on the implants and the grafted bone. Temporary restoration could be the major factor leading to failure in this case

1.12 Conclusion

Bone grafting procedure is often needed to be performed prior to implant placement. Modern technique, instrument, biomaterial, and better understanding of bone biology increase the success rate of this procedure. Several important factors when using this procedures are the following:

- Use only evidence-based technique.
- Good planning. Planning includes surgical and prosthetic planning. Implant should only be inserted in the correct 3-D position.
- Stay minimally invasive. Avoid any surgical procedure as possible. Also reduce the number of surgical procedure. This can reduce patient's morbidity.
- Use only biomaterial with a good scientific documentation.
- Patient selection. Not every patient is suitable for this procedure. Bone grafting procedure is associated with more time-consuming, more patient's morbidity, possible complication, and more cost.
- Technique selection. Every physician should choose which technique and biomaterial are suitable. One technique that works good in one doctor might not be suitable for others.

References

1. Cawood JI, Stoelinga PJ. International research group on reconstructive preprosthetic surgery. Consensus report. Int J Oral Maxillofac Surg. 2000;29:159.
2. Cawood JI, Howell RA. A classification of the edentulous jaws. Int J Oral Maxillofac Surg. 1998;17:232.
3. Neukam FW, Hausamen JE, Scheller H. Möglichkeiten und Grenzen der Implantologie beim älteren Patienten. Dtsch Zahnärztl Z. 1989;44:490.
4. de-Freitas NR, Lima LB, de-Moura MB, Veloso-Guedes CC, Simamoto-Júnior PC, de-Magalhães D. Bisphosphonate treatment and dental implants: A systematic review. Med Oral Patol Oral Cir Bucal. 2016;21(5):e644–51.
5. Khoury F, Hidajat H. Extensive autogenous bone augmentation and implantation in patients under bisphosphonate treatment: a 15 case series. Int J Periodontics Restorative Dent. 2016;36(1):9–18.
6. Chen ST, Buser D. Implants in post extraction sites. Literature update. In: Buser D, Belser U, Wismeijer D, editors. ITI treatment guide, vol. 3. Basel: ITI; 2008. p. 9–16.
7. Deporter D, Watson P, Pharoah M, Todescan R, Tomlinson G. Ten year result of a prospective study using porous surfaced dental implants and a mandibular overdenture. Clin Implant Dent Relat Res. 2002;4:183–9.
8. Fugazotto PA. Shorter implants in clinical practice: rationale and treatments results. Int J Oral Maxillofac Implants. 2008;23:487–96.
9. Misch CE, Steignga J, Barboza E, Misch Dietsh F, Cianciola LJ, Kazor C. Short dental implants in posterior partial edentulism: a multicenter retrospective 6 year case series study. J Periodontol. 2006;77:1340–7.
10. Feldman S, Boitel N, Weng D, Kohles SS, Stach RM. Five year survival distributions of short length (10 mm or less) machined surface and osseotite implants. Clin Implant Dent Relat Res. 2004;6:12–23.
11. Buser D, Dula K, Hirt HP, Belser U. Localized ridge augmentation with autograft and barrier membrane. Periodontol. 1999;19:151–63.
12. Buser D, Dula K, Belser U, Hirt HP, Berthold H. Localized ridge augmentation using guided bone regeneration. Surgical procedure in maxilla. Int J Periodontics Restorative Dent. 1993;13:29–45.
13. Isbaner J. Membranen in der zahnmedizin. Jahrb Implantol. 2016;2016:277.

Mandibular Bone Graft

2

Andi Setiawan Budihardja

Intraoral autogenous bone is a prime source for donor bone graft. The bone from the intraoral region not only has osteogenic, osteoconductive, and osteoinductive graft properties; in addition, the cortical bony structure has the benefit of mechanical resistance properties. Intraoral donors can be used to reconstruct alveolar bone defects from the horizontal, vertical, or a combination of the two [1, 2].

Intraoral cortical bone structure is better equipped to resist bone resorption when compared with bone from extraoral (iliac) sites. This is a major advantage to harvesting grafts from intraoral bone. However, the small volume of intraoral bone available for harvesting limits the cases in which intraoral grafting can be utilized to reconstructions with small to moderate bone defects. Grafts may be obtained in the form of:

- Monocortical bone graft (both cortical and cancellous bone).
- Cancellous bone only.

Intraoral autogenous bone grafts can be obtained from the symphysis mandible, retromolar (ramus) region, anterior sinus wall, maxillary tuberosity, edentulous region, mandibular tori, and crista zygomaticoalveolaris. The use of bone collectors that attach to the salivary suction is not recommended due to high bacterial contamination.

In general, large volume of bone can be obtained from the retromolar and symphysis regions, while other intraoral sites offer very limited amounts [2–4]. Grafts from the mandibular symphysis offer both cortical and cancellous bone properties in the greatest volume. This is advantageous with regard to graft healing; however, if not done carefully, harvesting from this region frequently results in sensitivity and

A. S. Budihardja (✉)
Department of Oral and Maxillofacial Surgery, Faculty of Medicine, University Pelita Harapan, Jakarta, Indonesia

Siloam Hospital Lippo Village, Jakarta, Indonesia

Budihardja Dental Specialist Center, Jakarta, Indonesia

A. S. Budihardja, T. Mücke (eds.), *Bone Management in Dental Implantology*,
https://doi.org/10.1007/978-3-319-78951-4_2

vitality problem of the adjacent teeth [5]. In addition, it requires two layers of mucosal suturing to avoid dehiscence and infection. It is recommended to do the lateral cephalometric x-ray or CBCT before harvesting the bone from the symphysis. As a result of the morbidity associated with this donor site, the symphysis is not the first choice for intraoral grafting.

Retromolar bone has very limited cancellous bone properties. Therefore, it is not ideal to promote bone healing and graft regeneration. Several studies have demonstrated large amount of non-vital osteocytes in this type of bone (until the third year), which undermines the osseointegration process [6]. For this reason, it is strongly recommended to improve osteoconductivity if using retromolar grafts.

	Retromolar	Symphysis
Bone structure	More cortical bone, limited cancellous	Cortical and cancellous bone
Volume	Less	More
Complications	Injury to n. alveolaris inferior Risk of mandible fracture	Sensory alterations to anterior teeth Damage to anterior teeth
Field of operation	Narrow operating field	Larger operating field Easy access
Limitation	– Wisdom tooth can limit the bone that can be harvested – Severe atrophic jaw increases the risk of jaw fracture	Long root, especially the canine

Osteoconductive is defined as the ability of the graft to serve as a scaffold for osteoblasts. Osteoblasts can penetrate via two mechanisms: (1) neovascularization from recipient region and (2) ability to recruit osteoblasts from the surrounding bone tissue [6, 7]. The osteoconductive process can be promoted by increasing the area/volume of the graft itself. For example, block grafts have lower osteoconductive properties in comparison with particulate graft, because the latter has a larger surface area. A study by Pallesen et al. [8] indicates that regeneration is accelerated in cases which utilized smaller graft particles (0.5–2.0 mm^3) as opposed to large (10 mm^3) after 2 and 4 weeks. Several techniques, such as Khoury's autogenous bone shell technique, can increase the osteoconductivity potential of the graft and reduce the risk of graft loss due to insufficient graft particulate stability [7].

The maximum volume that can be obtained from the retromolar region is 4.4 cm^3, while the symphysis is 4.8 cm^3. This can be done by utilizing special instruments (e.g., microsaw or piezosurgical tools). In contrast, using conventional techniques will result in significantly reduced volume obtained [9–11]. A study performed by Misch showed that osteotomies performed with a fissure bur resulted in maximal volumes of only 0.9 cm^3 from the ramus and 1.74 cm^3 from the chin [12]. Postoperative complications include sensitivity problem on chin area, ptosis of the chin, and patient aesthetic profile when the bone is harvested from this area [13, 14] (Figs. 2.1, 2.2, and 2.3).

	Piezosurgery	Microsaw	Lindemann bur	Bone scraper/trephine bur
Volume	Large	Large	Less	Medium
Tissue trauma	Minimal	Minimal	More trauma	Considerable
Operating time	Lengthy	Fast	Fast	Fast
Handling	Good	Good	Good	Good
Cost	Expensive	Average	Inexpensive	Average

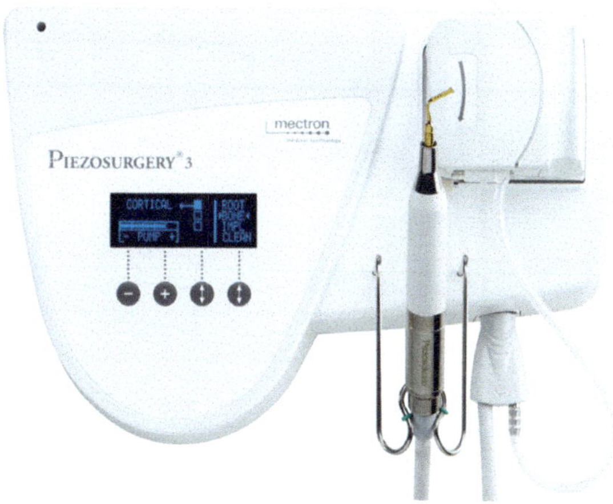

Fig. 2.1 Piezosurgery device and microsaw can be used to harvest great amount of autogenous bone from the mandible with less trauma

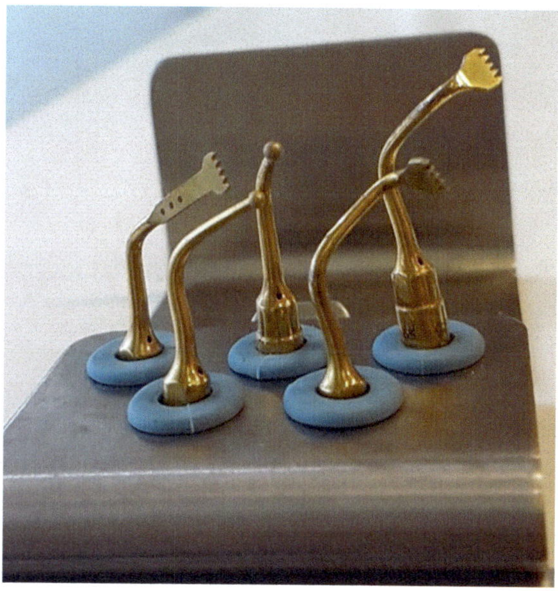

Fig. 2.2 Various tip for piezosurgery device

2.1 Indication

Intraoral bone reconstruction with autogenous mandibular bone without any membrane is indicated in the case where there are moderate to severe defects in the maxilla or mandible. In this situation it is not possible to insert dental implant in correct 3D position with primary stability. It is also useful in the case where previous surgery with artificial or alloplastic material has failed. If there is still possibility to insert dental implant in correct 3D position with primary stability, the author would recommend to use more minimal invasive technique such as guided bone regeneration technique (Fig. 2.4).

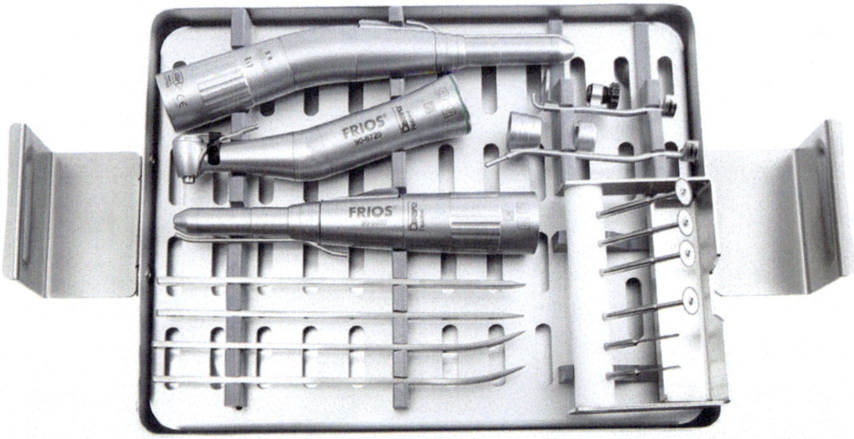

Fig. 2.3 Complete set of microsaw for bone harvesting (Invented by Prof. F. Khoury). Piezosurgery device and microsaw can be used to harvest great amount of autogenous bone from the mandible with less trauma

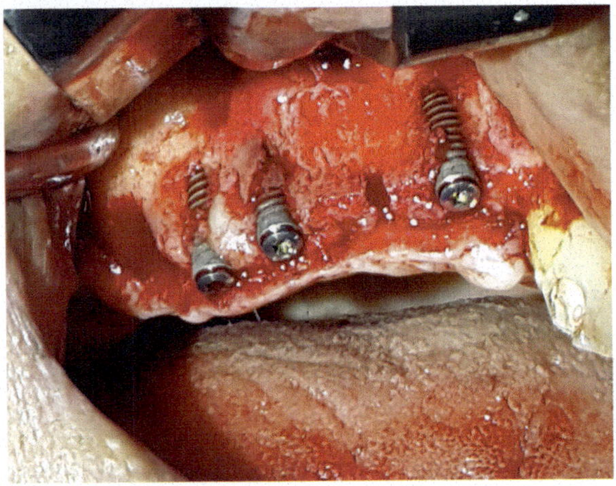

Fig. 2.4 If dental implant can be inserted in correct 3D position with primary stability, guided bone regeneration technique using membrane is preferable to augment the bone

2.2 Patient Preparation

Prior to surgery, a careful history, clinical examination, laboratory, and radiological workup are necessary, to ensure there are no contraindications to surgery. Radiographic examinations include orthopantomogram (OPG), lateral cephalometric, and cone beam computed tomography (CBCT). Planning can be done manually or with utilization of auxiliary software to ensure more accurate results in borderline and complex cases. CBCT should have a strong and clear indication, since it exposes the patient to considerable radiation. Every radiographic examination has to follow the ALARA (as low as reasonably achievable) principle.

Surgery may be performed under general anesthesia or local anesthesia with sedation (e.g., midazolam). Complex surgery under general anesthesia is usually performed in hospital and typically reserved for complex cases with an estimated operating time of three or more hours, with a possibility of more blood loss. Penicillin-group antibiotics, with clavulanic acid, are administered 1 h prior to surgery. In case of penicillin allergy, patients can be treated with clindamycin. Antibiotics should be continued for 5–7 days postoperatively. Provision of antibiotics with a rational dose is recommended, as prolonged antibiotic use has no correlation with favorable surgical outcomes and often results in bacterial resistance. Analgesic medications are also administered 1 h prior to surgery and continued for 7 days, in accordance with the patient's needs. Ibuprofen is usually sufficient for pain relief in bone graft operations; it can be also combined with paracetamol. In addition, chlorhexidine mouthwash should be used three times daily for 1 week postoperatively.

2.3 Surgical Technique of Harvesting Bone from the Ramus

The operation can be performed under local anesthesia, namely, buccal and lingual infiltration using 4% articaine with 1:100,000 epinephrine. Inferior alveolar nerve blocks are not recommended, because they allow no warning on proximity of the osteotomy to the nerve, often resulting in injury. The opening trapezium incision is similar to that used in a classical third molar osteotomy. A mucoperiosteal flap is reflected, exposing the bone at the external oblique ridge and lateral aspect of the ramus. Two Langenbeck retractors are used to protect the soft tissue. Osteotomy is performed on the proximal vertical aspect, baso horizontal and occlusal. Osteotomy is then performed to the outer cortex of the ramus area and is continued until it meets the cancellous area to prevent injury to the underlying neurovascular bundle. This is usually known when bleeding from the cancellous bone occurs. Medially the border of the osteotomy is the mesial root of the second molar.

Devices used for osteotomy include Lindemann bur, microsaw (Fig. 2.5), trephine bur (Fig. 2.6), and piezosurgery (Fig. 2.7a–c). Benefit of using microsaw is the ability to safely perform osteotomy in deep regions, with minimal trauma,

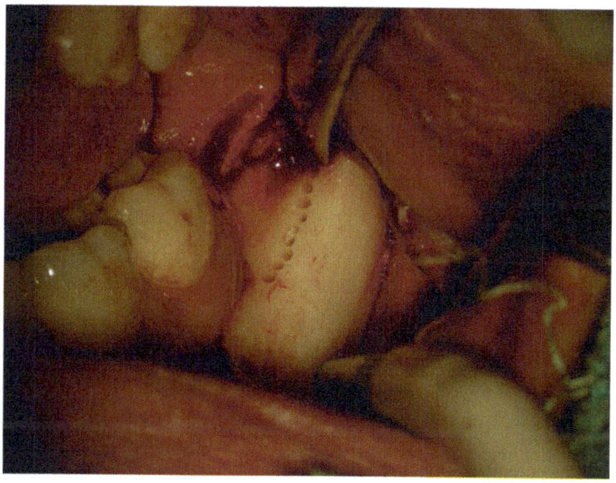

Fig. 2.5 Bone harvesting from the ramus using microsaw

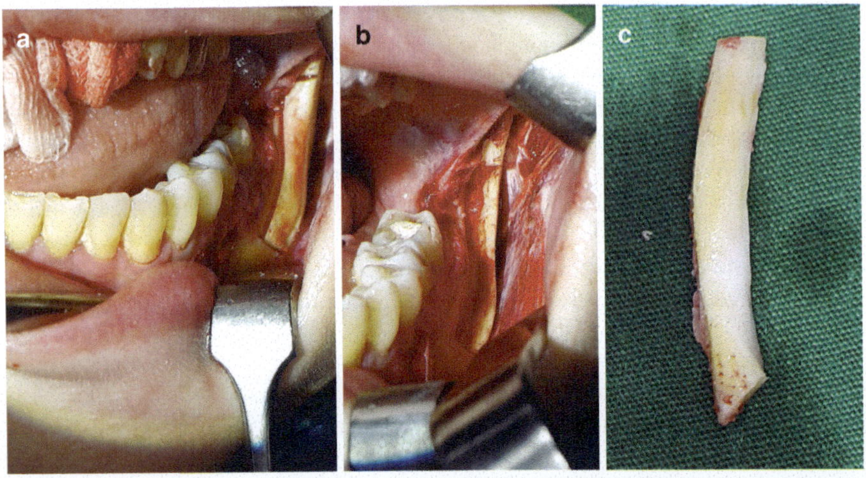

Fig. 2.6 (a–c) Bone harvesting from retromolar area using piezosurgery device

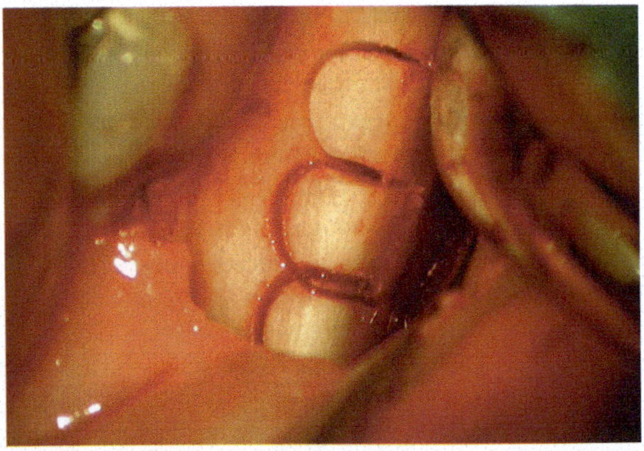

Fig. 2.7 Harvesting bone from retromolar area using trephine bur

thereby reducing unnecessary bone loss [15, 16]. Piezosurgery also is advantageous, allowing minimal trauma and preservation of nerve integrity. This method, however, is more time-consuming and results in longer surgical procedures.

Following osteotomy, a chisel can be used to gently remove the graft from the ramus. Bleeding can be controlled with bone wax (using only as much as necessary) and bipolar coagulation. The donor area is treated with collagen dressing for local hemostasis and promotion of wound healing and then closed with a 4.0 suture.

The bone block is then prepared for the recipient site, reshaped, and contoured in accordance with its requirements. A retromolar bone block may be split into two thin blocks with the use of a microsaw. Once the desired shape is achieved, the graft is positioned for fixation. Each bone block should ideally be fixated with two titanium miniscrews (diameter 1.0 or 1.2 mm). The operator must practice extreme caution

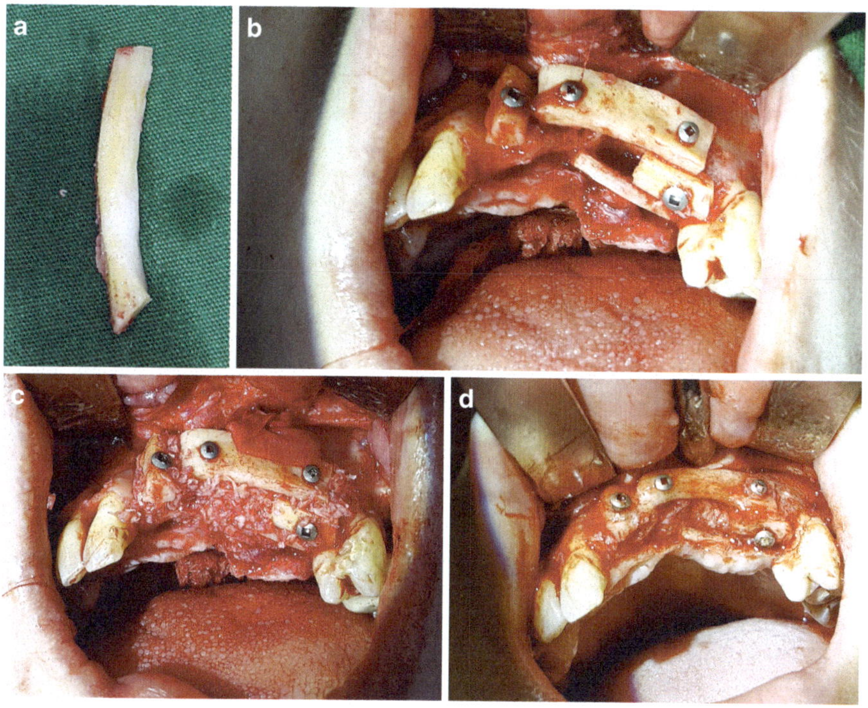

Fig. 2.8 (**a**–**d**) Autogenous mandibular bone was used to reconstruct vertical and horizontal defect in the anterior maxilla. The bone block was fixated on the buccal and palatal aspect. The gap between bone plate on the buccal and palatal area was filled using autogenous particulate bone. No membrane was used in this technique. Dental implants can be inserted 4 months after bone grafting procedure

when using fixation screws, so as not to injure the roots of neighboring teeth. Any sharp angles in the bone block that could perforate the soft tissue should be trimmed

Bone blocks can be fixated either in the form of a single monocortical block or using Khoury's 3D and bone shell technique (both buccal and lingual side are reconstructed using bone block), in which a gap is left between the cortical bone graft and the recipient site, which is then filled with cancellous bone (Fig. 2.8a–d). This technique allows for greater osteoconductivity of the graft ([7]). No alloplastic bone graft or other biomaterial is needed to fill the gap. Closure of the autograft material with membrane is not necessary since it can increase the rate of the dehiscence.

Tension-free closure of the soft tissues can be facilitated by a careful periosteal releasing incision. This can be done on buccal and lingual side. Failure of the operator to achieve tension-free closure can result in dehiscence, increasing the likelihood of graft failure. In case of big defect augmentation, it is necessary to do papilla shifting suturing technique. Closure of the mucosa is performed with 3.0 and 4.0 PTFE sutures. Use of sutures smaller than 5.0 in the critical area is not recommended. Sutures may be removed after 7–10 days postoperative.

Patients are encouraged to apply cold compresses for the first 2 days following surgery and to eat a soft diet for 2 weeks. Oral hygiene is advised, with regular brushing and chlorhexidine mouth rinse.

Generally, the healing period of the graft is approximately 4 months, after which dental implants may be placed. Titanium screws must be removed before placement of the dental implants, so as not to impede on the implant position. Dental implant placement is performed as usual.

2.4 Surgical Technique of Harvesting Bone from Mandibular Symphysis

The operation can be performed with local anesthesia, namely, buccal and lingual infiltration. An oblique incision is made, taking care to consider the location of mental foramen, so as not to injure the nerve. The mental nerve and root apices bilaterally should then be identified. Identification of the mental nerve bilaterally is mandatory in all operations in the symphysis region. The osteotomy may be performed by utilizing several different surgical tools, such as the Lindemann bur, microsaw, or piezosurgery (Fig. 2.9a, b). Because of the anterior loop of the mental nerve, it is crucial to stay at least 5 mm anterior of the mental foramen and at least 3 mm inferior to root apices. A chisel may then be used to remove the bone. Adequate control over bleeding is necessary to reduce postoperative hematoma. Hemostasis can be managed using bone wax and bipolar coagulation. Because bone wax is not resorbed, conservative usage is recommended, using the minimal amount necessary.

Several alternative methods may be used to fill bony defects, namely:

- Left alone, filled with frozen blood.
- Fill with collagen preparation, with or without membrane.
- Alloplastic bone grafts, closed with membrane.

Wound closure should be completed in two layers. The periosteum may be sutured with 4–0 resorbable suture, followed by the superficial mucosa, using 5–0 monofilament suture. Sutures may be removed on day 10 postoperative. The use of bandages on the chin for 5 days is recommended to reduce swelling and hematoma.

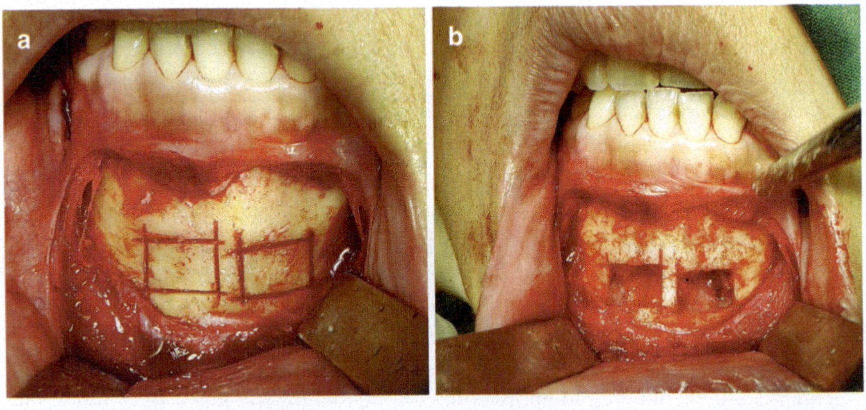

Fig. 2.9 (**a**, **b**) Harvesting two bone blocks from symphysis area using piezosurgery device

The following steps in management are identical to that of bone harvesting from the ramus.

2.5 Surgical Technique of Bone Harvesting from Torus Mandible

Autograft can also be harvested from the torus (mandible or palatal) or from other edentulous mandible (Fig. 2.10a–e). Operation can be performed under local anesthesia. Subperiosteal preparation of the flap is very important to protect important structure if one raises the lingual flap. Osteotomy can be done using piezosurgery

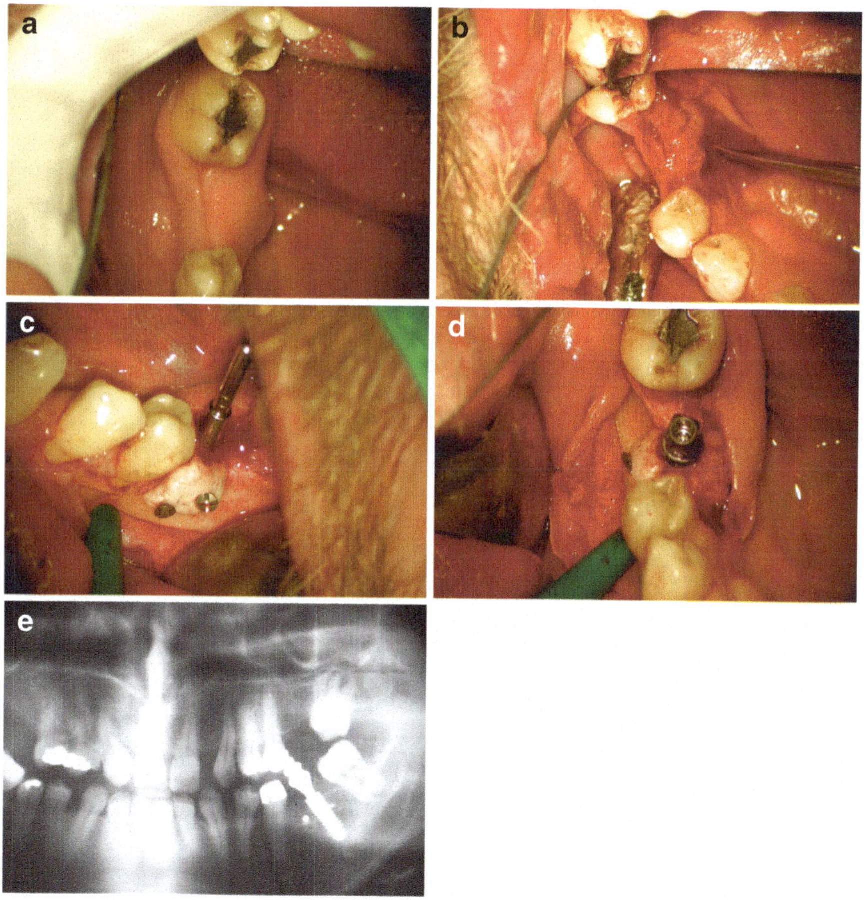

Fig. 2.10 (**a**–**e**) Horizontal bone defect was reconstructed using autogenous bone that was harvested from torus area. This can reduce patient's morbidity because it is not needed to harvest bone from the other area. Dental implant was inserted 4 months after with good primary stability. Good formation of the bone was seen around dental implant

device. The bone block is then luxated using a chisel. Bleeding can be controlled using bone wax and bipolar coagulation. The wound is sutured using 4.0 or 5.0 suture material.

Note must be taken that the bone harvested from the torus has low regenerative properties. It is advisable to combine it with cancellous bone or bone substituting osteoconductive material.

2.6 Harvesting Bone Using Bone Scraper

A large amount of cancellous bone can be harvested using bone scraper instrument (Fig. 2.11a, b). After harvesting monocortical bone block from the retromolar area or from symphysis area, cancellous bone is visible. This can be harvested using bone scraper instrument. Cancellous bone that can be harvested is enough to do bilateral sinus augmentation or moderate bone graft. It can be used to fill the gap between the original bone and grafted bone.

The bone that is harvested can be used solely as an autograft or it can be mixed with alloplastic bone graft material.

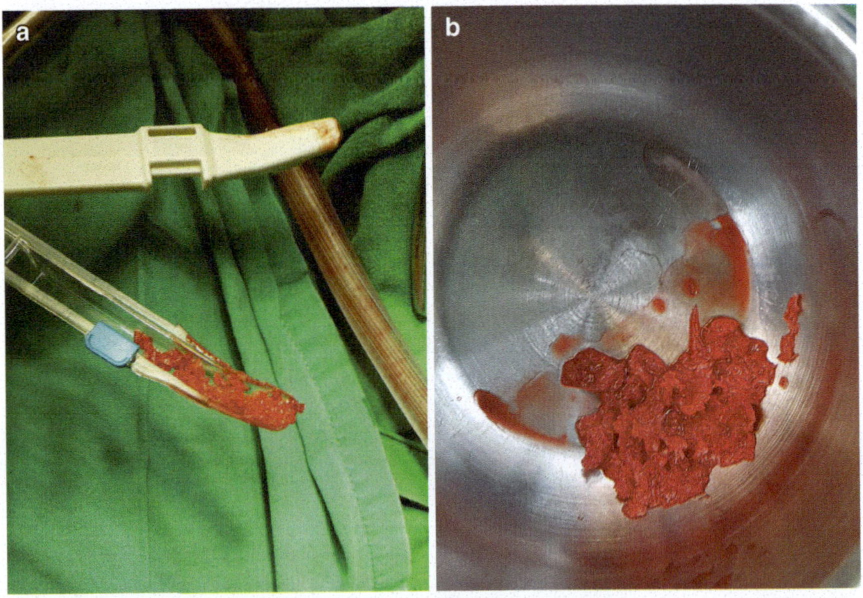

Fig. 2.11 (**a**, **b**) Cancellous bone was harvested using bone scraper

2.6.1 Representative Case No. 1 (Figs. 2.12a–i and 2.13a–h)

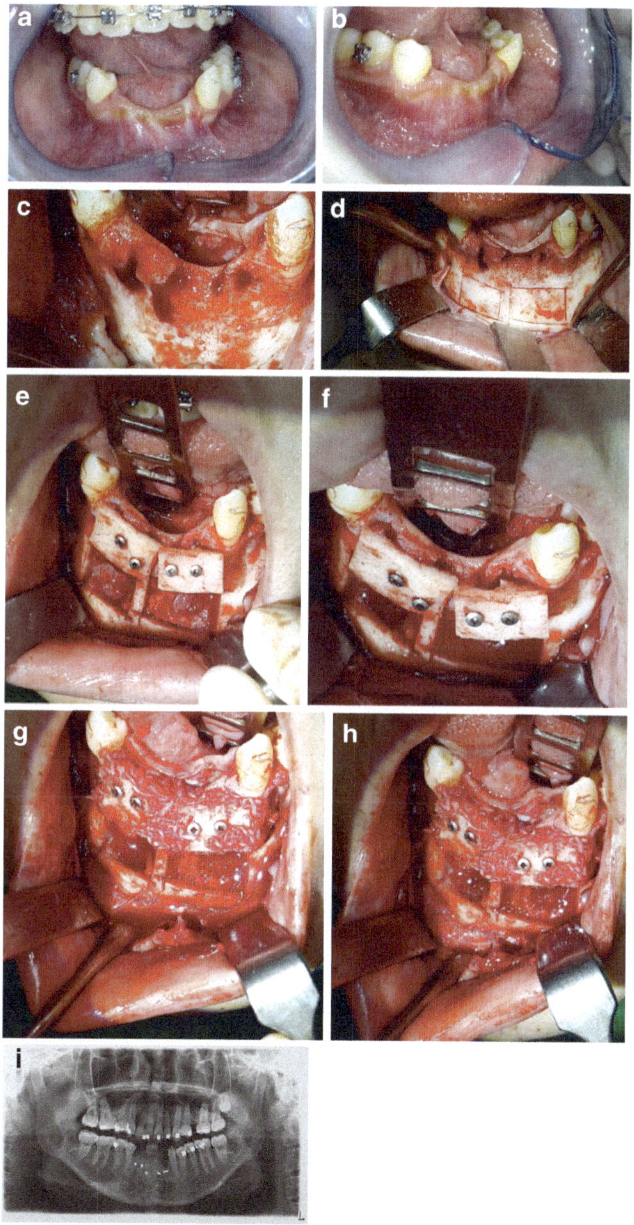

Fig. 2.12 (**a–i**) Horizontal and vertical bone defect in the anterior mandible after treatment of the mandible fracture 1 year before. Fracture of the mandible was treated with oral rigid internal fixation (ORIF) using miniplate titanium. These plates were then removed 1 year after the surgery. Bone defect was reconstructed using two autogenous bone blocks that were harvested from symphysis area. Bone blocks were fixated using 1.2× 11 mm miniscrew titanium to the original bone from a distance, leaving empty space between the original bone and harvested bone. This gap was filled with autogenous bone particle. No membrane or other biomaterial was used

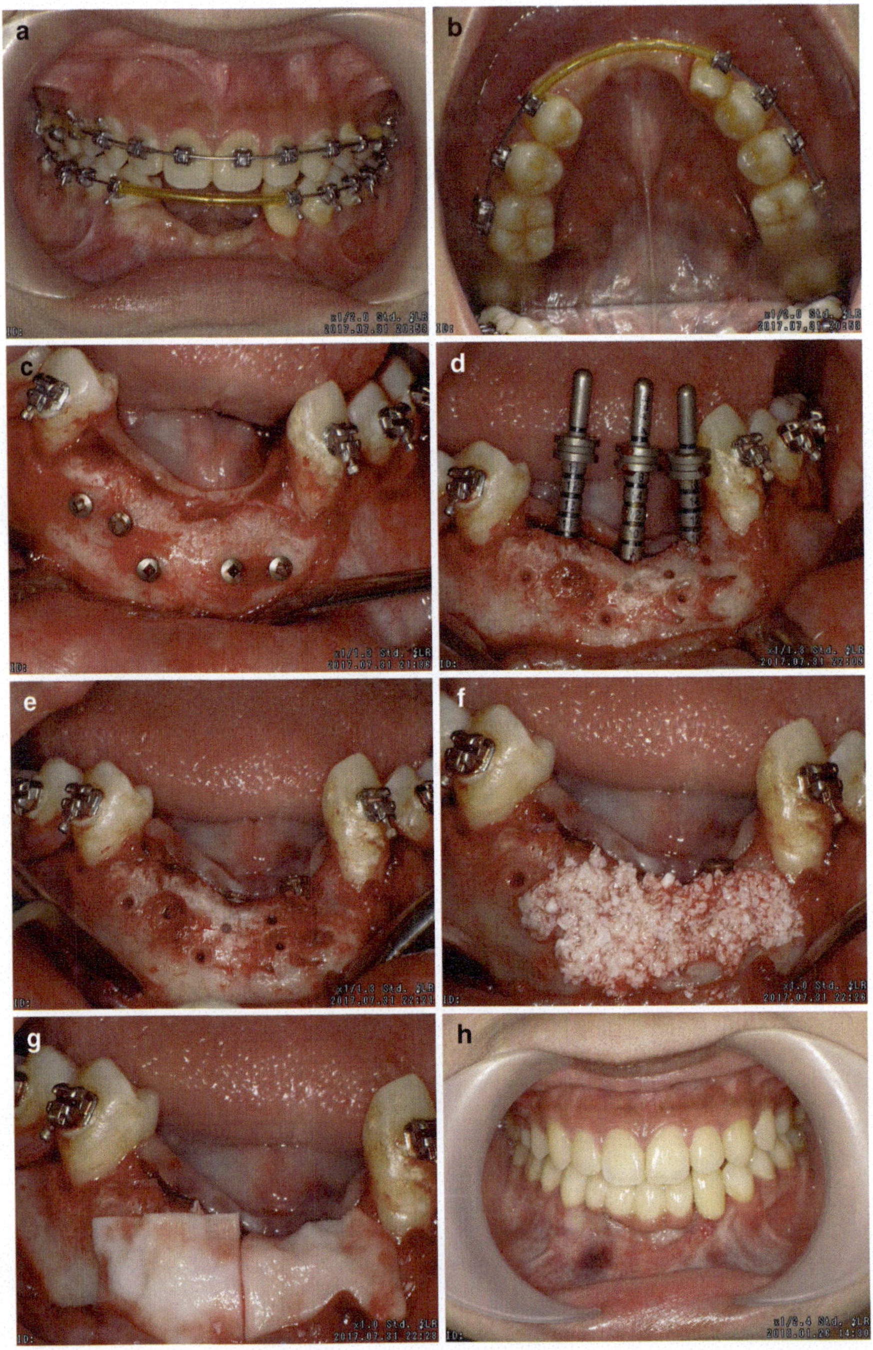

Fig. 2.13 (**a**–**h**) 5 months following uneventful healing, the site was reopened. Good vital bone formation was visible; this allowed three dental implants to be inserted in correct 3D position. To optimize the ridge contour, the facial bone was once more augmented with GBR technique using autogenous bone + ABBM particle and resorbable membrane. Prosthetic restoration can be done 3 months after (Prosthetic restoration by Dr. Devi Budihardja, Jakarta, Indonesia)

2.6.2 Representative Case No. 2 (Figs. 2.14a–d and 2.15a–i)

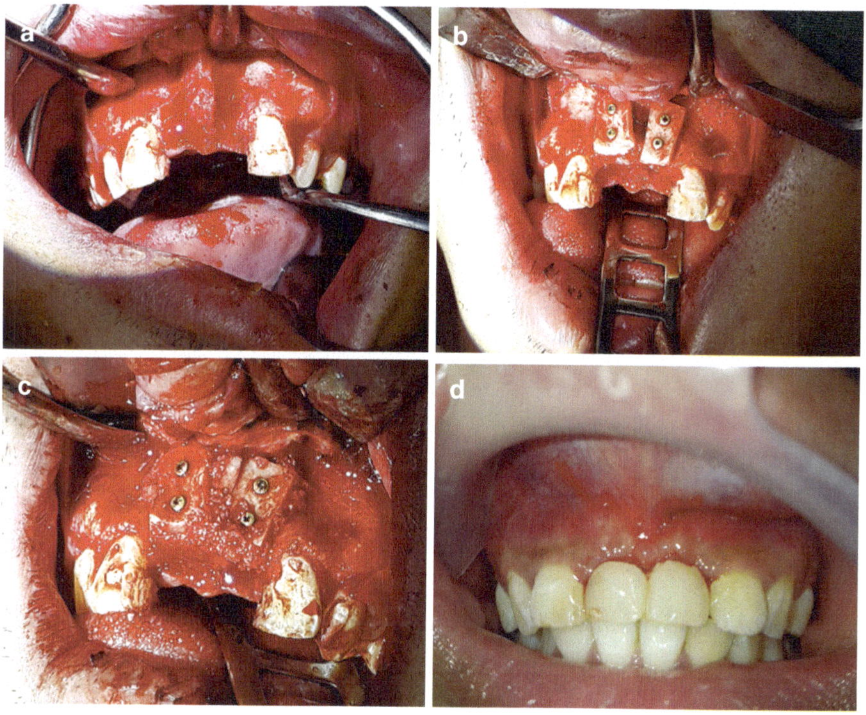

Fig. 2.14 (**a–d**) Patient presented with severe bone loss on regions 11 and 21 following history of dentoalveolar trauma 10 years ago and multiple failed endodontic treatment. Horizontal and vertical bone defect was reconstructed using two bone blocks. The bone was fixated using 1.2 × 12 mm titanium screw. The gap between the original bone and transplanted bone was filled using only autograft. No membrane or other biomaterial was used in this case. Tension-free soft tissue closure is achieved using periosteal incision and shifting one papilla suture. Temporary restoration using Maryland bridge. There must be no pressure on the grafted bone during the healing period

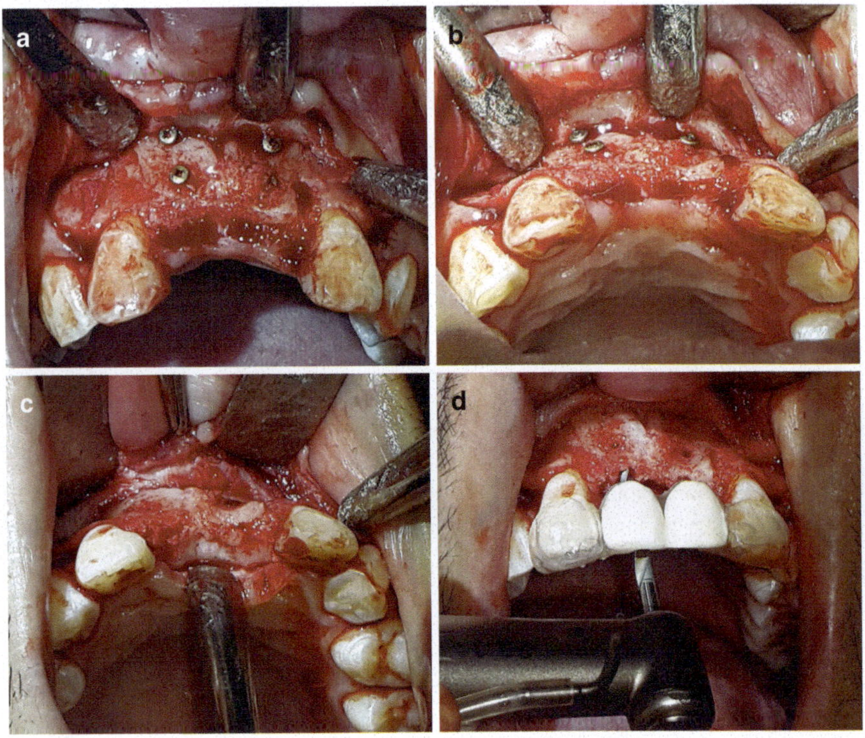

Fig. 2.15 (**a–i**) Site reentry after 4 months healing period. Sufficient amount of healthy bone was visible. Dental implants were inserted in correct 3D position. All implants have primary stability with good soft tissue around implants. Definitive prosthetic restoration after 5 years shows a stable bone and soft tissue around implants

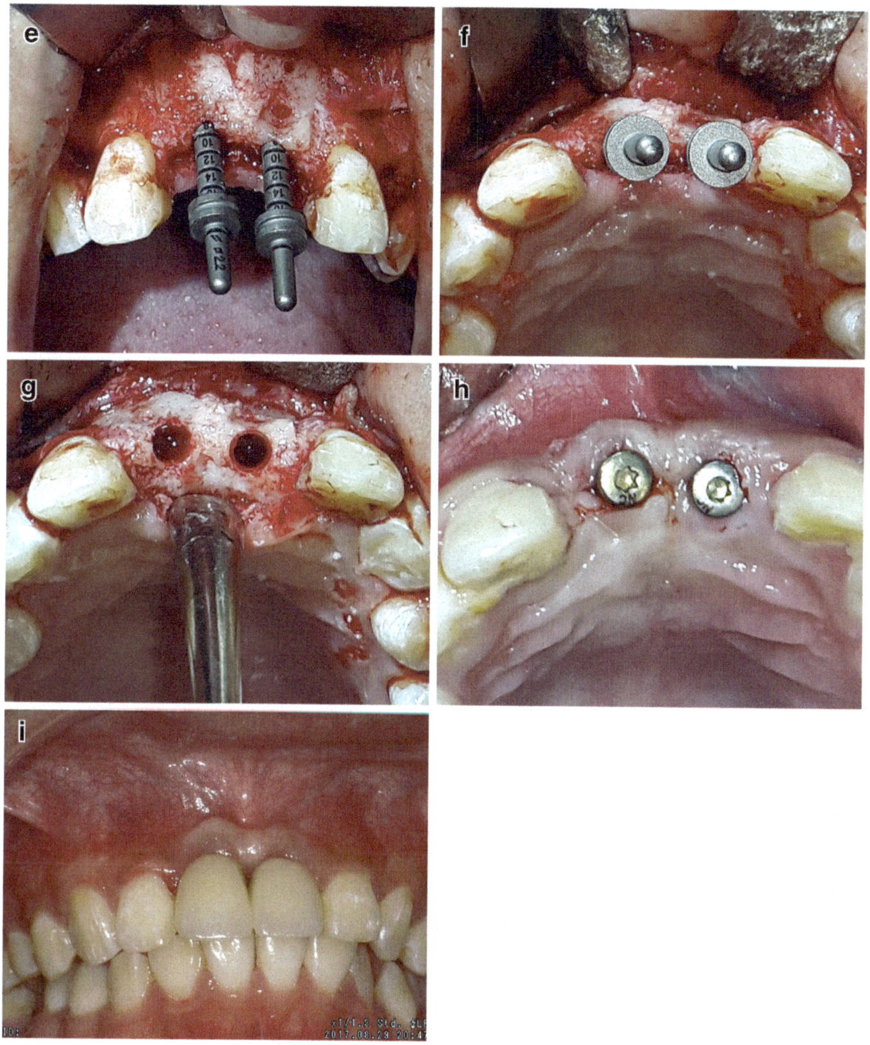

Fig. 2.15 (continued)

2.7 Conclusion

Reconstruction of severe atrophic jaw presents a challenge. Vertical bone reconstruction is in general more difficult and more unpredictable than horizontal bone reconstruction. Bone grafts from intraoral donor sites can be used to perform reconstruction on small to moderate bony defects. The bone from retromolar area is an excellent donor site for this purpose. Cortical and cancellous bone can be harvested from this area.

The use of a donor from the symphysis is necessary if multiple cancellous bones are required. The success rate of donor use from intraoral is very high, if performed by experienced operators with the proper technique.

Mandibular bone graft can be used for the treatment of horizontal and vertical bone defect. Advantages using mandibular bone graft are:

- No need to use any membrane to cover graft material, since the cortical bone of the mandibular bone graft can serve as a membrane to protect graft material from the invasion of the soft tissue ingrowth.
- Minimize the risk of graft exposure because no membrane is needed.
- Easier to close the soft tissue without tension.
- No need to use any alloplastic biomaterial, thus can reduce the risk of infection and rejection and can also reduce the cost.
- Shorten treatment time. In general a 4-month healing time is recommended before implant can be inserted.
- Better bone quality when only autogenous bone is used.

The use of special instrument such as microsaw and piezosurgery is very useful, allowing operators to perform operations quickly, precisely, and atraumatically, so as to minimize complications during and after surgery.

Good surgical techniques, careful tissue handling, as well as knowledge of anatomical structures are essential to support the successful outcome of this procedure.

Disadvantages using this technique include the donor site morbidity and it requires high skill and experience from the operator.

References

1. Clementini M, Morlupi A, Agrestini S, Ottria L. Success rate of dental implants inserted in autologous bone graft regenerated area: a systematic review. Oral Implantol. 2012;4:3–10.
2. Neukam FW, Mosgau SS. Implantate bei ausgedehnten Knochendefiziten. In: Koeck B, Wagner W, editors. Implantologie ed; 2004. p. 200–15.
3. Proussaefs P, Lozada J, Kleinman A, Rohrer MD. The use of ramus autogenous block graft for vertical alveolar ridge augmentation and implant placement: a pilot study. Int J Oral Maxillofac Implants. 2002;17:238–48.
4. Zouhary KJ. Bone graft harvesting from distant sites: concept and technique. Oral Maxillofac Surg Clin North Am. 2010;3:301–16.
5. Nkenke E, Schultze Mosgau S, Radespiel Tröger M, Kloss F, Neukam FW. Morbidity of harvesting chin grafts: a prospective study. Clin Oral Implants Res. 2001;12:495–502.
6. Günzl HJ, Khoury F. Morphologische Untersuchungen von Knochenbiopsien nach autogener Alveolar Extensionsplastik am unentkalkten, kunststoffeingebetteten Schlifpräparat. In Gesselschaft für orale Implantologie. Jahrb Orale Implantol. 1993;153.
7. Khoury F, Khoury C. Mandibular bone block grafts: diagnosis, instrumentation, harvesting technique and surgical procedure. In: Khoury F, et al., editors. Bone augmentation in oral implantology. Surrey: Quintessence; 2007. p. 116–35.
8. Pallesen L, Schou s AM, Hjorting Hansen E, Nattestad A, Melsen F. Influence of particle size of autogenous bone grafts on early stage of bone regeneration: a histologic and stereologic study in rabbit calvarium. Int J Oral Maxillofac Implant. 2002;17:498–506.
9. Khoury F. Die modifizierte Alveolar extensionsplastik. Z Zahnärztl Implantol. 1987;3:174–8.

10. Khoury F. Chirurgische Aspekte und Ergebnisse zur Verbesserung des Knochenlagers vor Implantologischen Maßnahmen. Implant Dent. 1994;3:237–47.
11. Khoury F, Happe A. Zur Diagnostik und Methodik von Intraoralen Knochenentnahmen. Z Zahnärztl Implantol. 1999;15:167–76.
12. Misch CM, Misch CE, Resnik RR, Ismail YH. Reconstruction of maxillary alveolar defects with mandibular symphysis graft for dental implants: a preliminary procedural report. Int J Oral Maxillofac Implants. 1992;7:360–6.
13. Hunt DR, Jovanovic SA. Autogenous bone harvesting: a chin graft technique for particulate and monocortical bone blocks. Int J Periodontics Restorative Dent. 1999;19:165–73.
14. Montazem A, Valauri DV, St Hilaire H, Buchbinder D. The mandibular symphysis as a donor site in maxillofacial bone grafting: a quantitative anatomic study. J Oral Maxillofac Surg. 2000;58:1368–71.
15. Khoury F, Hemprich A, Sass T. Die Anwendung des freien Knochendeckels bei verschiedenen Eingriffen im Unterkiefer. Dtsch Z Mund Kiefer Gesichtschir. 1985;9:298–304.
16. Khoury F, Hensher R. The bony lid approach for the apical root resection of lower molars. Int J Oral Maxillofac Surg. 1987;16:166–70.

Guided Bone Regeneration, Bone Splitting, Interpositional Osteoplastic

3

Andi Setiawan Budihardja

3.1 Guided Bone Regeneration

Guided bone regeneration (GBR) refers to the procedure to guide bone growth at sites with insufficient dimension of bone. Guided bone regeneration is mainly indicated to correct horizontal bone deficiency. It can be done together with the dental implant insertion if dental implant can be inserted in correct 3D position with primary stability [1–3].

The main principle of GBR is using membrane to cover the osseous wound space from the ingrowth of the undesirably soft tissue. This will exclude osteogenic cells from the soft tissue, thereby allowing osteogenic cell to inhabit osseous wound without any interference. Vertical bone defect is shown to be very difficult and less predictable to be treated with GBR as shown in several publications. It is possible to reconstruct vertical defect with GBR using more stable membrane. Long term result still needed to know the success rate using GBR technique to treat vertical bone deficiency.

Guided bone regeneration can be carried out in two ways (Fig. 3.1a–g):

1. Two-step procedure. This means to first do the bone regeneration using GBR technique. After 4–9 months of healing period, dental implant can be inserted in the correct 3D position in the healing bone.
2. One-step procedure. This means dental implant can be inserted at the same time with the bone regeneration procedure. This can be done if dental implant can be inserted at the correct 3D position with primary stability and when primary soft tissue closure without tension is possible [4].

A. S. Budihardja (✉)
Department of Oral and Maxillofacial Surgery, Faculty of Medicine, University Pelita Harapan, Jakarta, Indonesia

Siloam Hospital Lippo Village, Jakarta, Indonesia

Budihardja Dental Specialist Center, Jakarta, Indonesia

A. S. Budihardja, T. Mücke (eds.), *Bone Management in Dental Implantology*,
https://doi.org/10.1007/978-3-319-78951-4_3

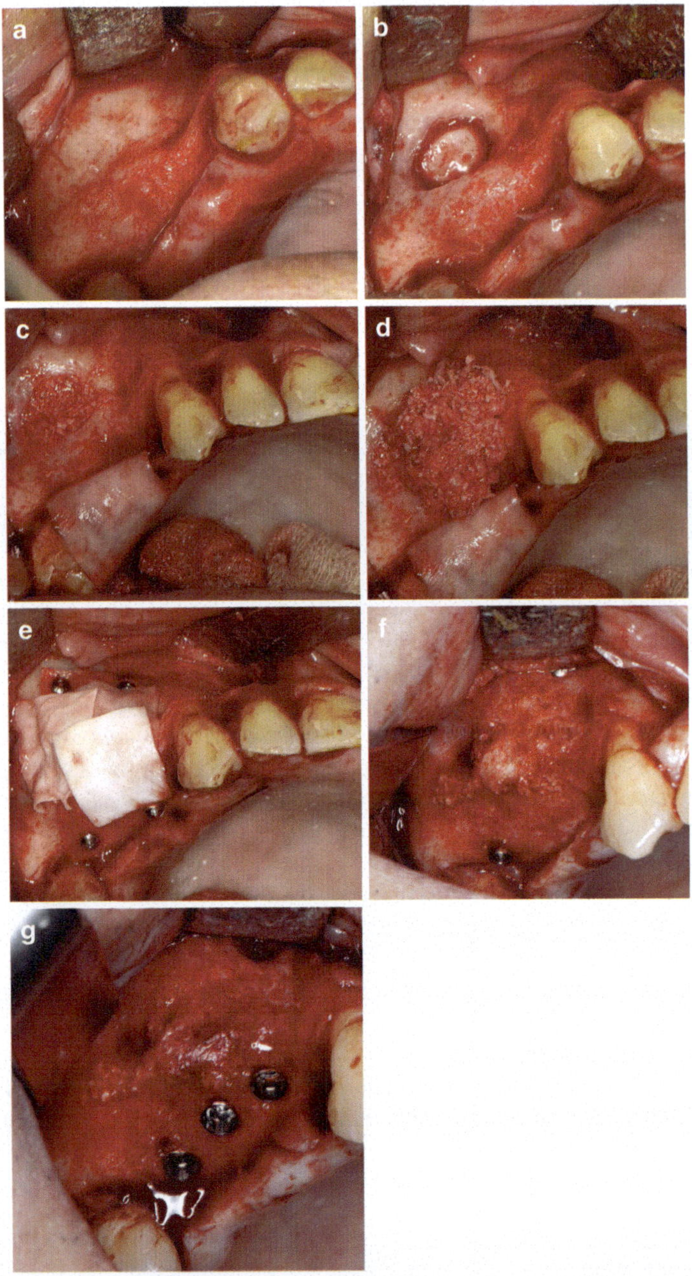

Fig. 3.1 (**a**–**g**) Horizontal bone defect on the maxillary regions 14–16 and vertical bone deficiency on regions 14–16. External sinus augmentation was done to correct vertical deficiency on the posterior maxilla, and two-step GBR procedure was done to correct horizontal bone deficiency on regions 14–16. Additional graft material (autogenous bone + ABBM) was placed on the buccal aspect to correct horizontal bone deficiency. Resorbable membrane was used to cover bone graft material. This membrane was fixed using small titanium pins. Another resorbable collagen membrane was used to cover the area that is not covered by the first membrane. Dental implant was inserted 6 months after bone grafting. Vital bone was shown on this area

Membrane functions in GBR [5–7]:

- To prevent cellular proliferation of soft tissue to bone graft area.
- Bone graft stabilisation.
- To avoid bone graft resorption by 25%.

Membranes should have the quality of biocompatibility (well accepted by the body), cell occlusivity (avoid soft tissue cell penetration into the defect), stability, and easy to use with licence (e.g. CE certification in Europe).

	Advantages	Disadvantages
Nonresorbable membrane • PTFE • ePTFE • ePTFE, titanium reinforced • titanium	• More stability • Longer barrier function • Can be used for more complex vertical and horizontal augmentation	• Second surgical procedure to remove membrane means larger wound incision at second stage surgery • Membrane exposure*
Resorbable membrane • Synthetic • Allogene • Bovine, porcine, equine	• No need membrane removal • Can be used for horizontal augmentation • Easy surgical handling • Faster vascularisation	• Membrane collapse • Shorter duration barrier function • Cannot be used for complex vertical augmentation*

*Expensive

Important qualities of resorbable membrane:

- Human body and bone graft biocompatible.
- Adequate barrier functions (at least 3 months) to protect bone graft from cellular proliferation.
- Good degradation time: Degradation can happen after bone regeneration around the implant.
- Not releasing antigen that can interfere healing process (especially in xenogenic membrane).

Important qualities of nonresorbable membrane (Fig. 3.2a–c):

- Easy to use and easy to be taken out.
- Human body and bone graft biocompatible.

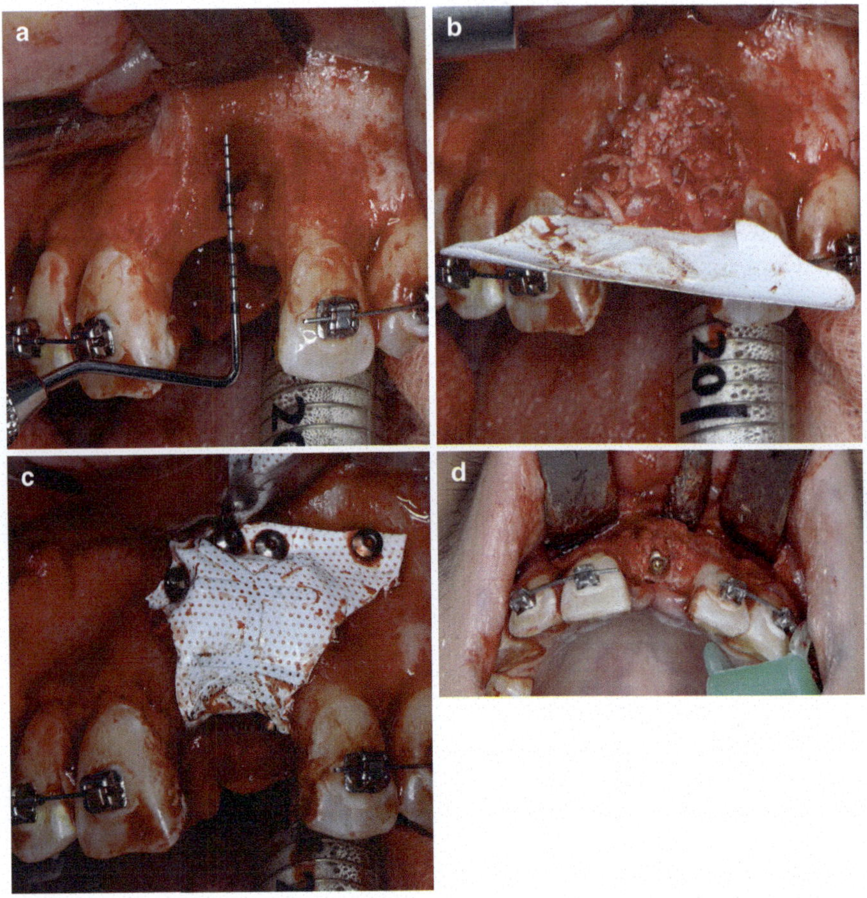

Fig. 3.2 (**a–d**) Guided bone regeneration using nonresorbable membrane was used to correct vertical and horizontal bone deficiency. The membrane was fixated using mini master pin on the buccal and palatal side. This membrane should be removed at the time of implant insertion 9 months after initial bone grafting surgery

3.2 Grafting Material

Autogenous bone is the "gold standard" material in any GBR procedure. Autogenous bone is the only material that has osteogenic, osteoconductive and osteoinductive properties. Moreover autogenous bone has mechanical property if the cortical bone is harvested in the block form. This osteogenic property is a crucial factor in bone regeneration. Using particulate bone is preferable than using block form. Particulate bone has more regenerative potential; this characteristic is related to the larger surface of the graft exposed to the growth factor. In GBR procedure, it is normally enough to harvest autogenous bone with bone scraper.

The use of alloplastic bone material, xenograft and allograft is also very common in GBR procedure. This material has osteoconductive potential. Combination of one of these materials with autogenous bone can be used in GBR technique. In two-step GBR procedure, this material can be mixed with autogenous bone. Most of the publications suggest to combine autogenous bone with osteoconductive bone graft material with the ratio 1:1; however, we find that using slightly more autogenous bone (around 70% autogenous bone) can increase bone quality resulting from this procedure.

3.3 Incision and Flap Design

Crestal incision is made across the length of the defect; vertical releasing incision is generally made one or tooth away from the defect. In simple GBR, one vertical releasing incision on the distal part of the defect is sufficient to close soft tissue without tension (Fig. 3.3). In the case where a large amount of bone grafting is needed on the large defect area, it is better to do two vertical two teeth away releasing incision. Two vertical releasing incisions facilitate easier flap closure without tension. There is no evidence that one vertical incision design is superior than the other; therefore, we always do simple straight vertical incision.

Vertical incision one tooth away from the defect on the palatal/lingual side is recommended to facilitate tension-free closure of the flap.

Flap should be sutured without tension; this can be achieved with gentle periosteal releasing incision on the buccal flap. Lingual flap also can be raised and careful periosteal releasing incision on the lingual side can be done to reduce tension. Dissection of the lingual flap should be done carefully with respect to important anatomical structure on the lingual side.

Wound closure can be done using 3.0 or 4.0 monofilament suture or PTFE suture material.

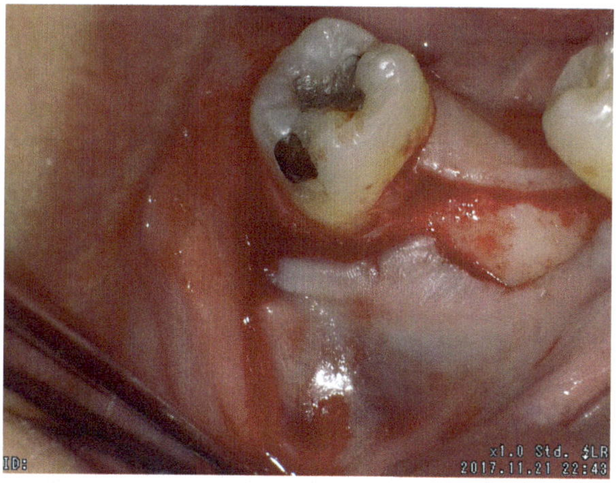

Fig. 3.3 One vertical releasing incision at the distal area usually enough to facilitate tension-free closure in the GBR procedure to reconstruct small to medium defect

3.4 GBR Operation Technique

In bone with thickness at least 5 mm, dental implants can be inserted with adequate primary stability but will create dehiscence in the buccal side. Operator should "create" this dehiscence in the buccal side, because guided bone regeneration is more difficult to do from the palatal side. Bone graft that is used can be from autogenous bone or mixed between autogenous and bone substituting material. Autogenous bone that is acquired from adjacent area with bone scraper is used to cover the exposed implants. Bone substituting material (BSM) is used to cover these autogenous bones and then the membrane on the top of it. Autogenous bone can also mixed directly with BSM and used to cover the defect [4, 8].

Membrane fixation is needed when using more stable membrane form, such as titanium membrane or ePTFE membrane; in some of the cases, fixation of resorbable membrane is also useful to provide more stable condition of the bone graft material. Fixation of the membrane is also needed when using resorbable membrane to do large horizontal augmentation. Read the manufacturer's instruction of

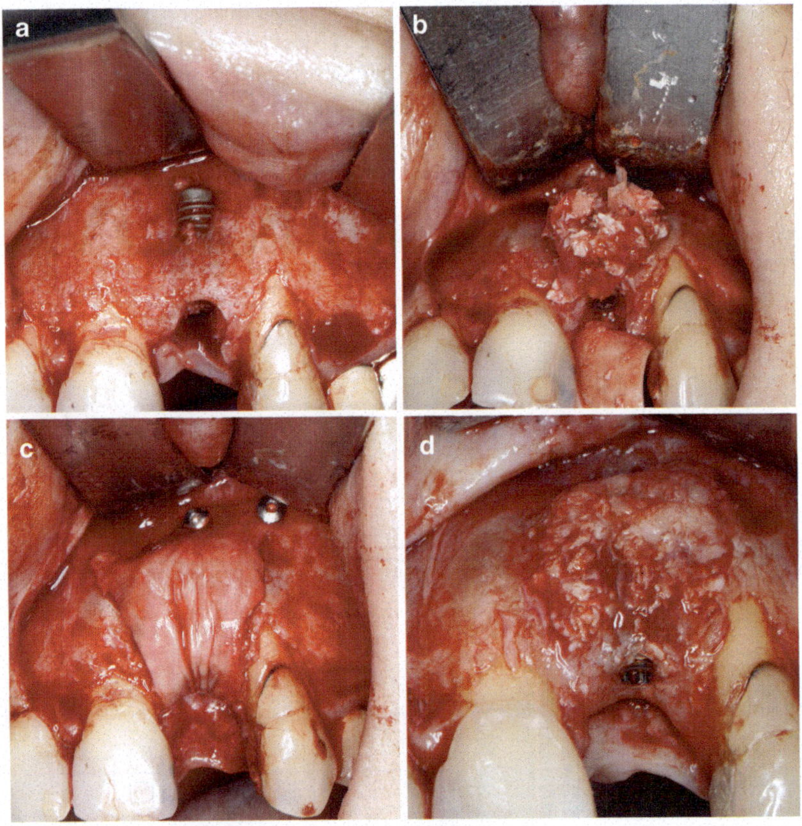

Fig. 3.4 (**a–c**) Dental implant was inserted with primary stability on the anterior maxilla. Guided bone regeneration using autogenous bone + ABBM was performed. Collagen membrane was fixated using small titanium pins. This is very important to maintain stability and volume of the bone graft material (**d**) 4 months after GBR procedure, second stage surgery was done. Vital and adequate bone could be seen on this area

each membrane used carefully; sometimes soaking the membrane in patient's blood is necessary [9, 10] (Fig. 3.4a–c).

Periosteum incision is done as needed to make sure that there is no tension in suturing the wound. Patient is given oral hygiene instruction including rinsing with chlorhexidine for 7 days. Oral antibiotic is given for 1 week postoperative.

3.4.1 Representative Case 1 (Fig. 3.5a–m)

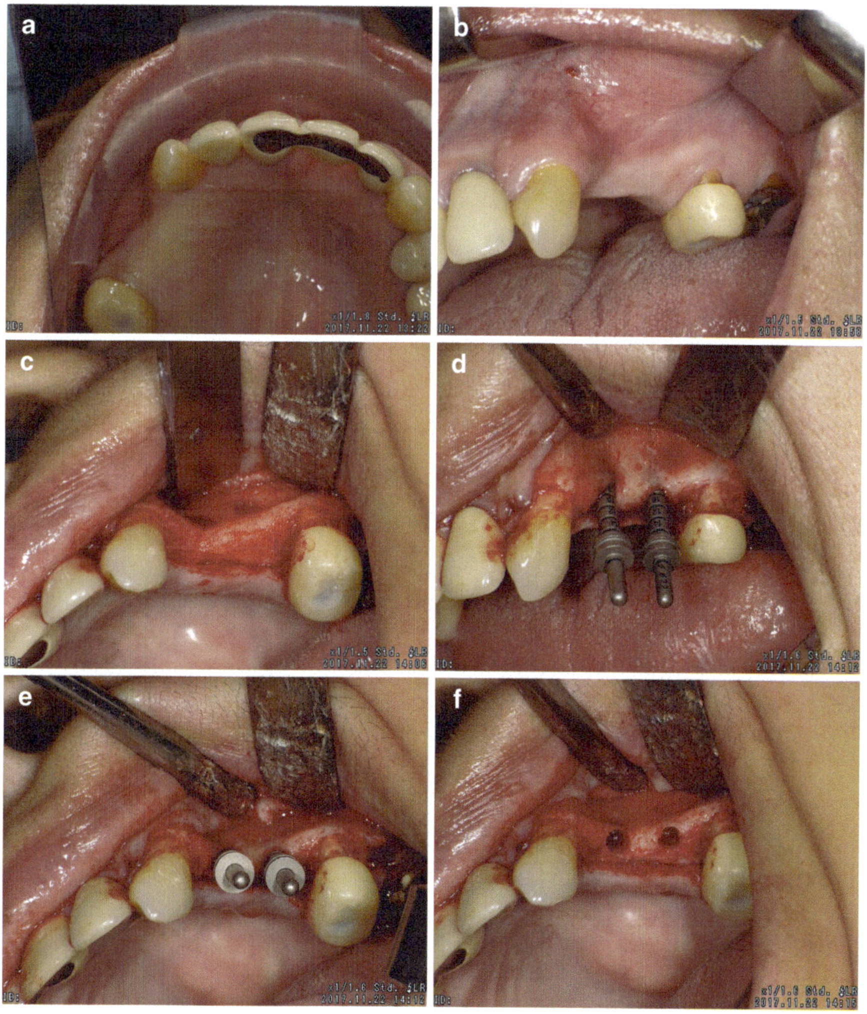

Fig. 3.5 (**a–m**) Horizontal bone deficiency on the posterior maxilla. Two dental implants were inserted in the correct 3D position with primary stability. GBR was performed using autogenous bone that was harvested with bone scraper; ABBM was applied on the buccal area. Double-layer collagen membrane was placed to cover the bone graft. Tension-free suture was done. In this case, it was enough to do only one vertical releasing incision

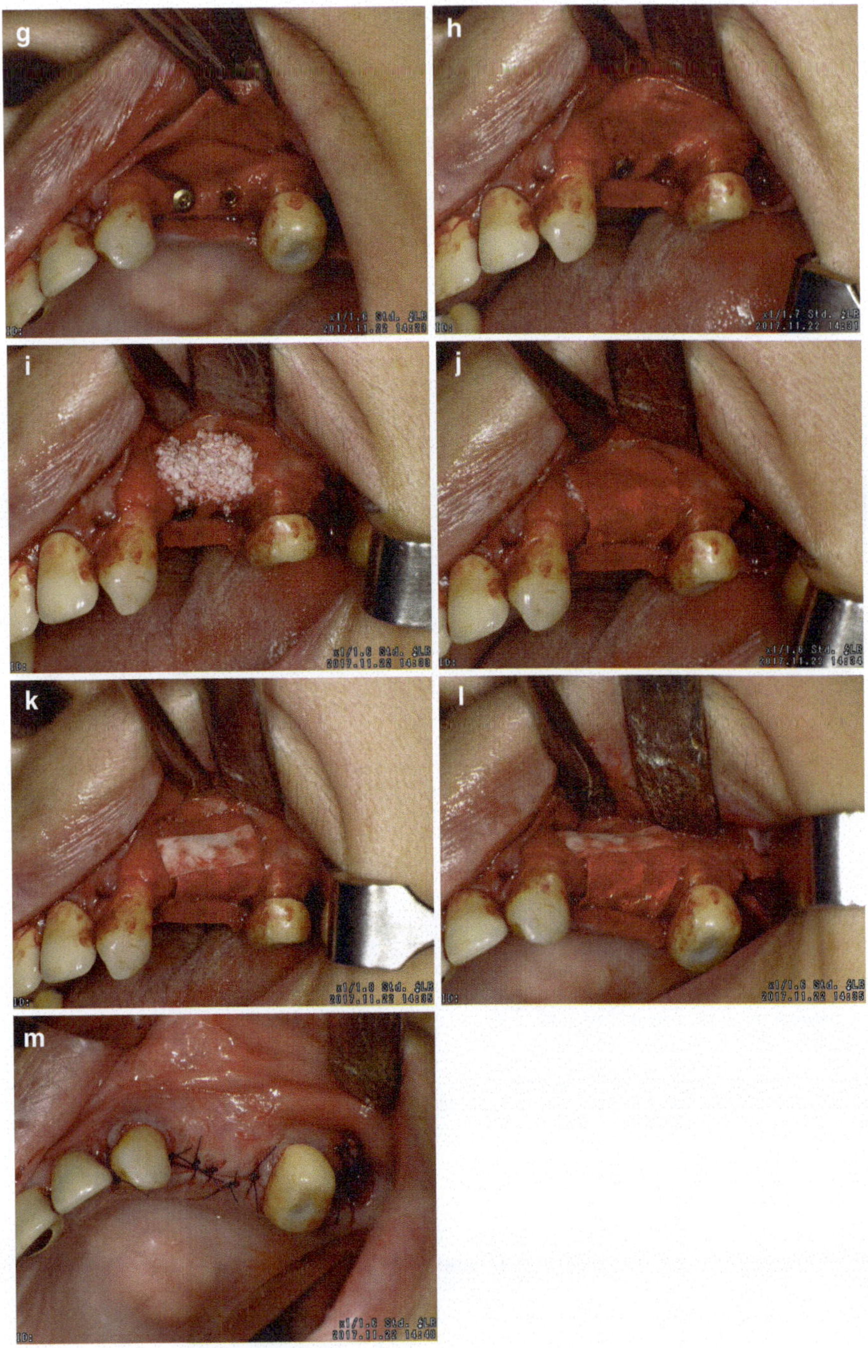

Fig. 3.5 (continued)

3.4.2 **Representative Case No. 3** (Figs. 3.6a–e and 3.7a–i)

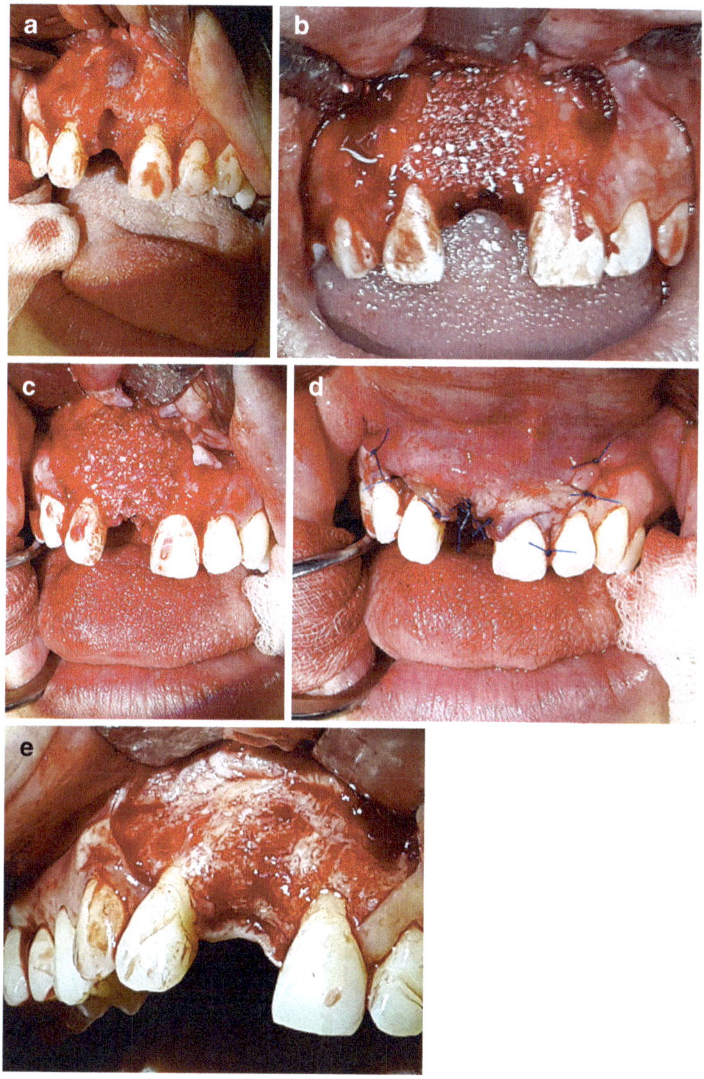

Fig. 3.6 (**a**–**e**) Tooth 11 was extracted, and cystectomy to remove periapical pathological tissue was performed. Histological examination revealed radicular cyst. Large bone defect after tooth extraction and cystectomy. It was not possible to insert dental implant in the correct 3D position with primary stability. Grafting the site using combination of autogenous bone and ABBM. Both materials were mixed 1:1 and then filled the gap. Double-layer collagen membrane was used to cover the graft. Periosteal incision was performed to ensure flap can be sutured without tension. Re-entry 4 months after GBR procedure. Good bone regeneration with adequate volume was observed. This makes dental implant insertion can be done easily

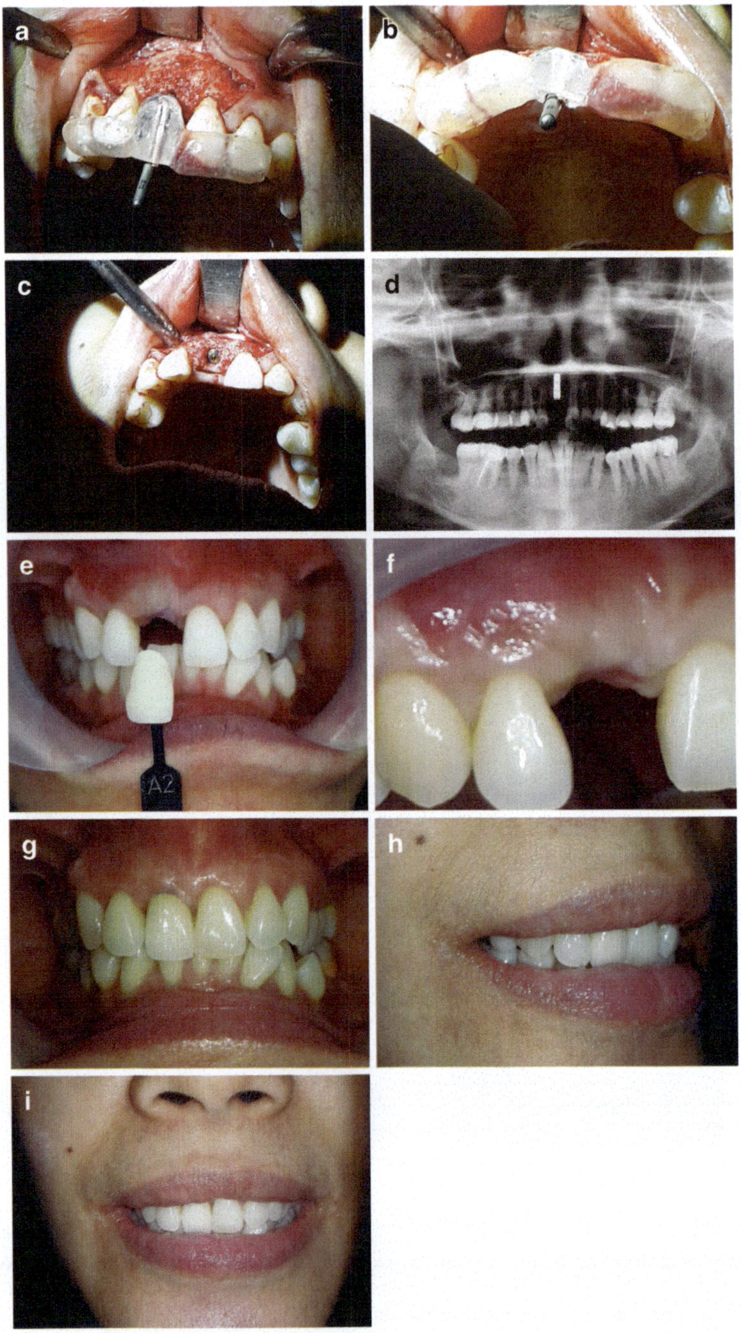

Fig. 3.7 (**a**–**i**) Dental implant was inserted with guidance from surgical template. It could be placed in the correct 3D position with primary stability. Four months after implant insertion, second stage surgery to place healing abutment was performed. Choosing the correct colour for the definitive restoration was done. Definitive crown restoration after 8 years in function shows stable periimplant bone and soft tissue (Prosthetic restoration by Dr. Devi Budihardja, Jakarta)

3.5 GBR Complication

The most common complication is infection. It is reported that bacteria such as *Staphylococcus aureus*, *Porphyromonas gingivalis*, *Bacteroides forsythus*, *Fusobacterium* and *Propionibacterium acnes* can colonise at the membrane, causing infection, membrane exposure and GBR failure (Fig. 3.8).

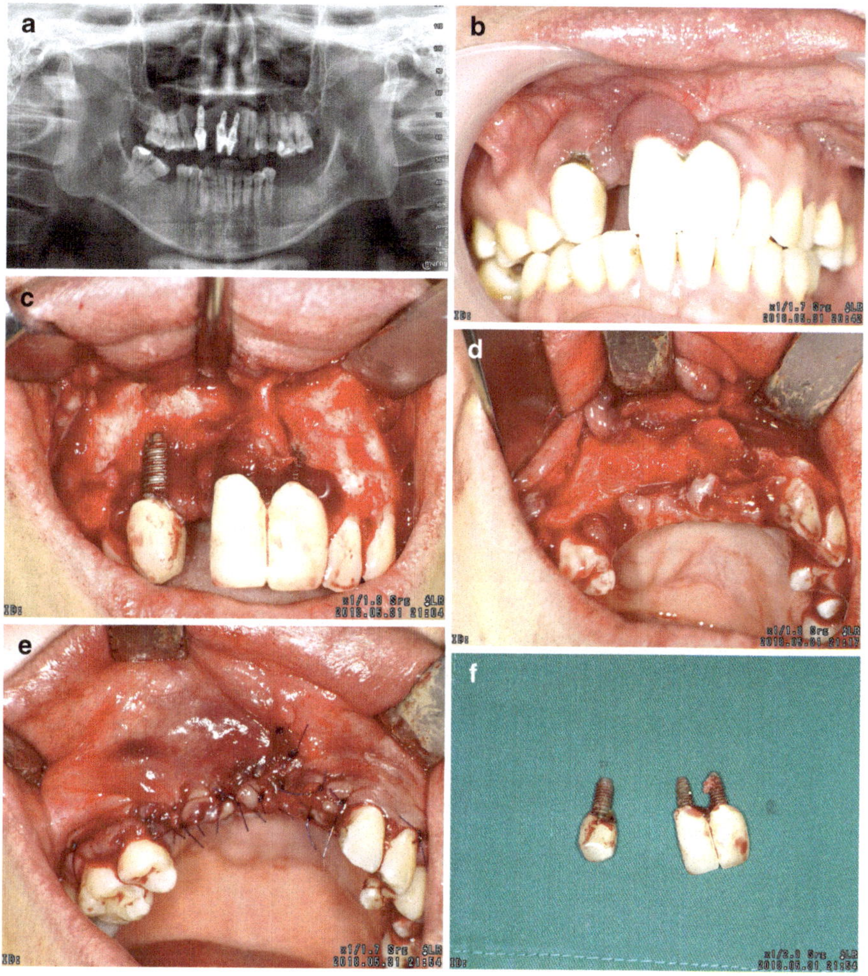

Fig. 3.8 (**a**–**f**) Patient reported four dental implants were inserted with additional bone graft procedure 1 year ago by her dentist. Few days after the surgery, the patient noticed that some bone graft materials were extruded to the nasal cavity. One dental implant was mobile and has been taken out 1 month after initial surgery. From the OPG can be seen three infected implants with severe bone loss. Multiple series of antibiotic was given to the patient without any improvement. We have then decided to remove all infected implants, remove all necrotic bone and close the soft tissue

Membrane exposure can also be caused by inadequate surgery procedure, failure to achieve tension-free closure, irritation from prosthesis (especially removable prosthesis) and host factor. It is not suggested to use removable prosthesis after GBR because it will create pressure on the graft. Rochette bridge can be used instead (Fig. 3.9a–k).

Host factor like uncontrolled diabetes mellitus, immune system-related disease, stress factor and smoking can amplify failure risk of GBR.

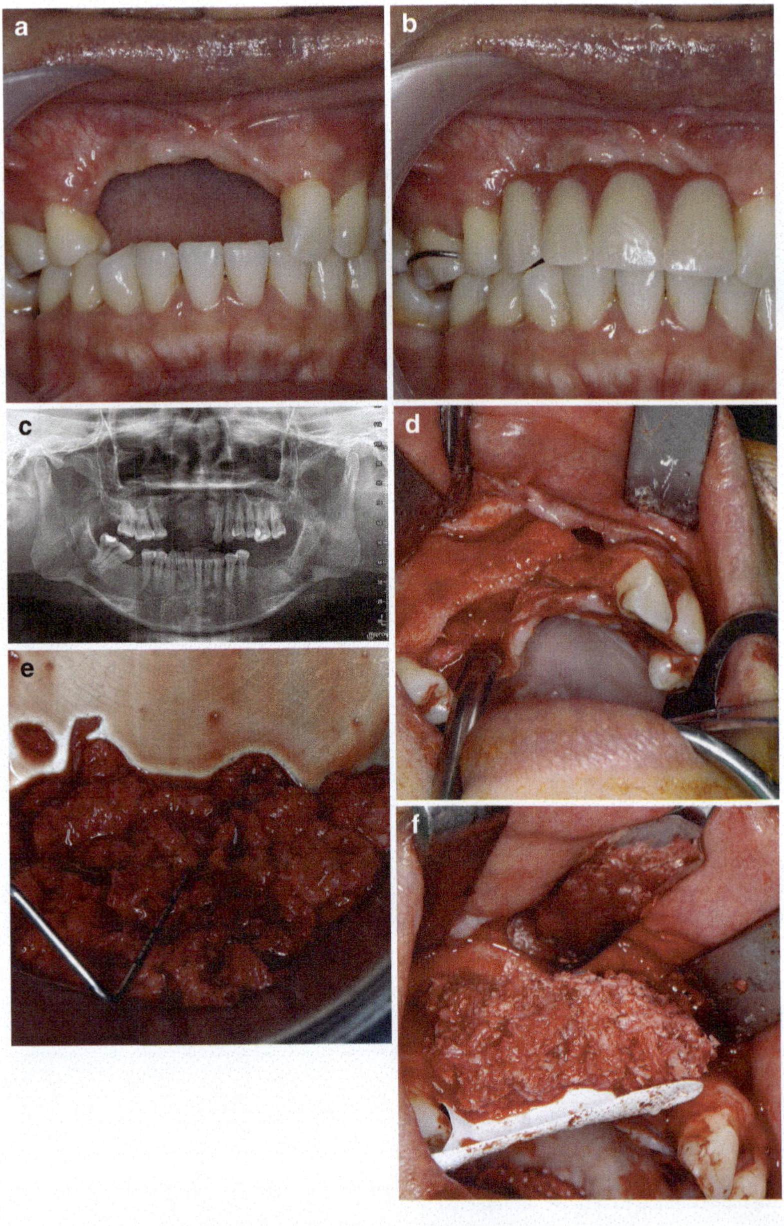

Fig. 3.9 (**a**–**k**) Intraoral situation 3 months after implant removal showed severe horizontal and vertical bone defect. Guided bone regeneration using autograft + ABBM and titanium-reinforced PTFE membrane was done to correct bone deficiency. Soft tissue closure was done after careful periosteal releasing incision. Postoperative X-ray shows good bone formation

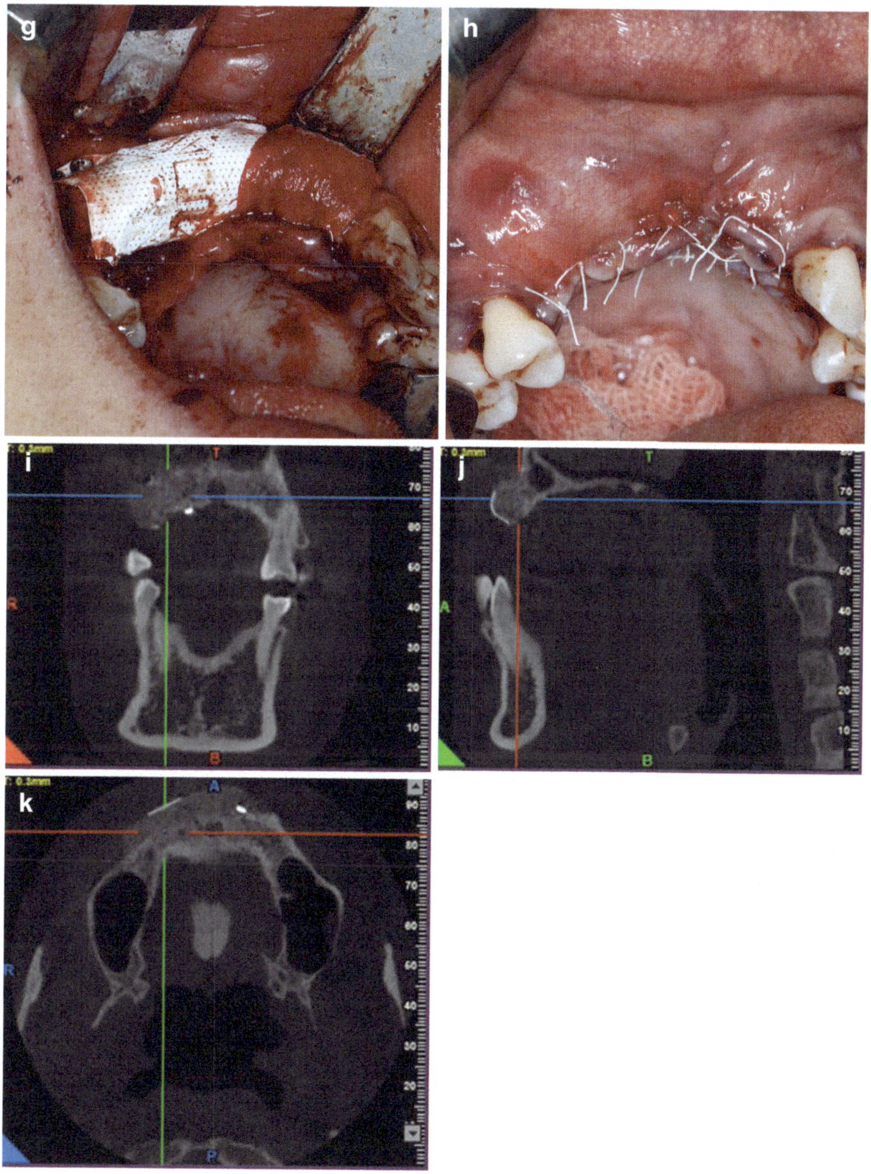

Fig. 3.9 (continued)

3.6 Conclusion

Guided bone regeneration is a well-established and well-documented procedure to correct horizontal and vertical bone deficiency. This technique has a very high success rate. It can be done in one-stage approach if dental implant can be inserted in the correct 3D position with primary stability and soft tissue can cover the wound without tension. It can also be done in two-stage approach, meaning dental implant can be inserted 4–9 months after GBR procedure.

Vertical defect is the most challenging defect to reconstruct using GBR procedure. Reconstruction of the vertical defect needs more stable membrane such as ePTFE membrane. Fixation of the membrane is very important in this procedure. It can be fixated using mini master titanium pin or using fixation suture.

Autogenous bone is gold standard material that should be used in any GBR procedure regardless of the technique or membrane that is being used. Graft material should consist of at least 50% of autogenous bone, 70 % is preferable.

Soft tissue closure without tension can be achieved with careful periosteal releasing incision on the buccal and lingual side. Advantages using GBR technique are: minimal invasive technique, easier to adapt bone graft in irregular bone contour and easy to apply the technique. Disadvantages of this technique are: longer healing time (6–9 months) comparing to mandibular bone graft (3–4 months) and costly procedure (need expensive membrane and other bone substituting material)

3.7 Bone Splitting

Bone splitting is indicated if the minimal bone thickness is 2 mm. This procedure is introduced by Nentwig and Kniha [11]. Under local anaesthesia, partial-thickness flap is done by letting the periosteum to be attached to the buccal bone to ensure sufficient blood supply. Osteotomy in alveolar crest is done with thin fissure bone, microsaw or piezosurgery. A thin chisel is used to create greenstick fracture of the buccal bone. Implant can be inserted directly if primary stability is achieved; if not then implant can be inserted after 3 months. Space between bones can be filled with autogenous bone or combination of autogenous bone and alloplastic bone graft material. Membrane is not necessary in this case. Flap can then be tightly closed with periosteum incision if needed.

Disadvantage in the use of this technique is that implant placement in the correct 3D position in most of the cases is not possible. In the anterior region, it can create aesthetic problem.

3.7.1 Representative Case No. 1 (Fig. 3.10a–e)

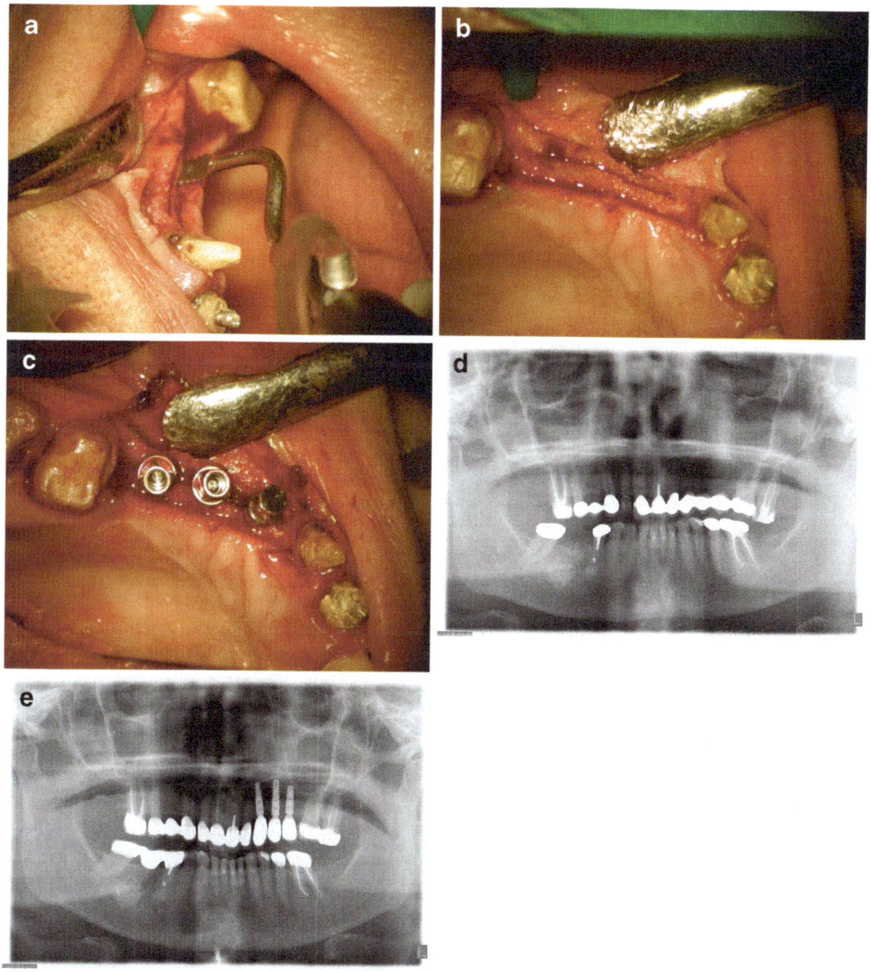

Fig. 3.10 (**a**–**e**) Bone splitting was done using ultrasonic device; this creates greenstick fracture. Dental implants were inserted; bony gap can be filled with combination of autograft and ABBM

3.7.2 Representative Case No. 2 (Fig. 3.11a–f)

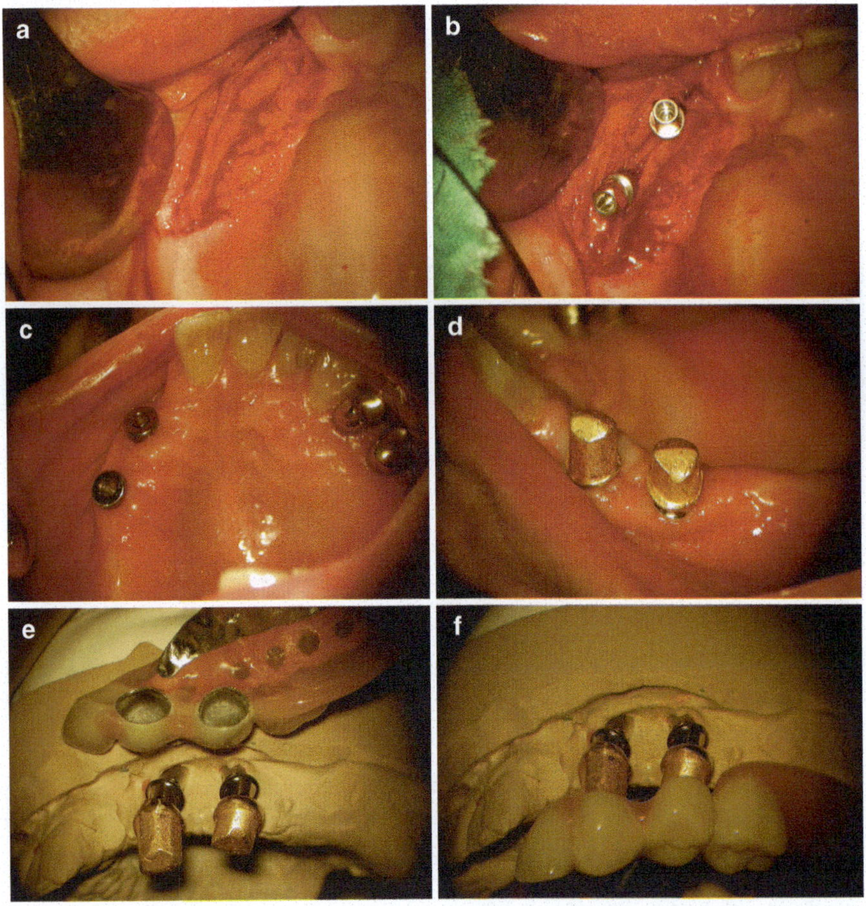

Fig. 3.11 (**a–f**) Thin bone on the posterior maxilla. Bone splitting with simultaneous dental implant insertion was done. Bony gap was filled with autograft and ABBM material. Prosthetic restoration using telescope removable denture (Case by Dr. Heiko Reese, Germany)

3.8 Interpositional Osteoplastic

Interpositional osteoplastic is used to enhance the height of alveolar bone (vertical area), especially at the mandible with severe resorption [12], where direct implant placement causes extremely long crown of the restoration.

Preparation for this procedure is just like other bone grafting procedures and can be done under local or general anaesthesia, starting with crestal incision, followed with mucoperiosteal dissection flap. It is important to identify left and right n. mentalis of the mandible. Osteotomy should be done at least 5 mm from foramen mentalis to avoid injury of the anterior loop of the n. mentalis.

Bone osteotomy is done with bone saw or piezosurgery on mesiovertical, distovertical and basohorizontal side. Bone fragment is then mobilised cranially with chisel. It is very important that the lingual bone is still intact with the periosteum. Temporary fixation can be done with miniplate 2.0 at the required bone height. Dental implant can then be inserted from crestal to the basal bone. Space in between two bone fragments can be filled with alloplastic material such as Norian SRS cement, as an alternative combination of autogenous bone + ABBM can be used to fill the gap; then two-layer wound closure is done using 4.0 and 5.0 monofilament suture material. Prosthetic restoration can be done after 4 months.

Norian SRS cement is a synthetic inorganic material, made of monocalcium phosphate, tricalcium phosphate, calcium carbonate and sodium phosphate. This material is usually used for maxillofacial defect reconstruction in sinus frontalis, nasoglabelar, supraorbital and mandible and can also be used on craniosynostosis and craniotomy defect. Norian SRS cement is biocompatible with the human body and has more compressive strength (4–10 times more) compared to cancellous bone (up to 50 MPa). Moreover, this material is osteoconductive and not osteoinductive.

Interpositional osteoplastic with Norian SRS cement has advantages such as reduce morbidity of the patient (no need to acquire bone from other body parts), reduce treatment time (distraction osteogenesis takes longer) and more comfortable for the patients. The disadvantage is that it needs high operator skill and backward planning so that the implant is placed according to the prosthodontic restoration.

3.8.1 **Representative Case** (Fig. 3.12a–g)

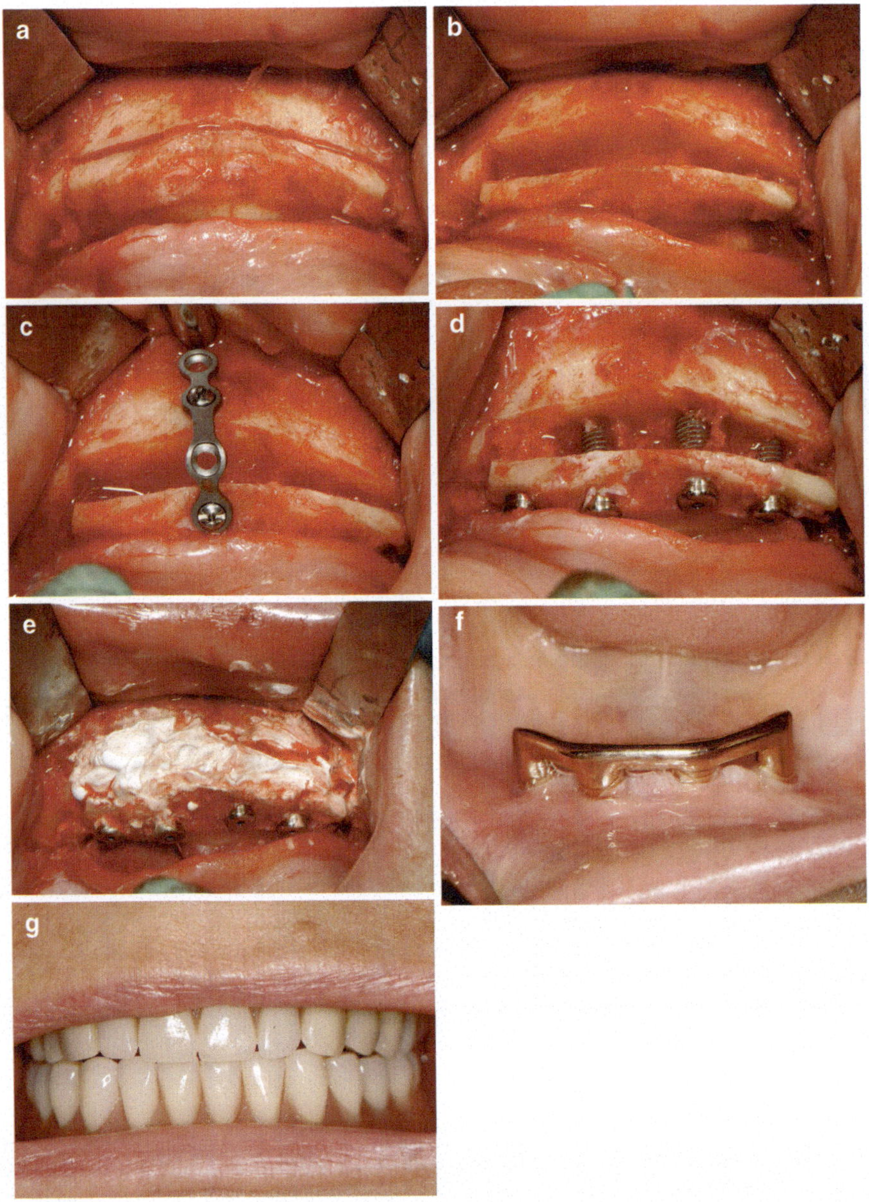

Fig. 3.12 (**a**–**g**) Osteotomy was done with microsaw, and as an alternative, piezosurgery also can be used. Bone fragment was moved to the cranial direction with the periosteum attached to the bony fragment. Temporary bone fixation in the desired place with 2.0 titanium miniplate system. Dental implants were inserted; the gap was filled with bone substituting material, and as an alternative autograft can also be used. Prosthetic restoration was performed 4 months after initial surgery

3.9 Conclusion

Interpositional osteoplastic is a very useful technique to correct vertical deficiency of the bone. Dental implant can be inserted at the same time with the IO procedure; this will reduce treatment time. In this case, we use Norian SRS cement material as a bone graft material. As an alternative, combination of autogenous bone and ABBM material can also be used.

Necrosis of the bone segment and fracture of the mandible are one of the major complications in using this technique. Periosteum on the lingual side must be attached to the bone to make sure that the vascularisation of the bone is adequate.

Disadvantage using this technique is that it is difficult to place dental implants in the correct 3D position; therefore, like in our case here, we use this technique mainly on the edentulous anterior mandible where the prosthesis restoration was done using hybrid denture.

This technique could be an alternative to the distraction osteogenesis. It does not need any expensive device and treatment time is shorter compared to distraction osteogenesis.

Credit: All surgeries in the subchapter interpositional osteoplastic were done at the Department of Oral and Maxillofacial-Plastic Surgery at Ruhr Universität Bochum, Germany, in the years 2001–2007 (Chairman: Prof. Dr. K. D. Wolff).

References

1. Buser D, Bornstein MM, Weber HP, Grutter L, Schmid B, Belser UC. Early implant placement with simultaneous guided bone regeneration following single tooth extraction in the esthetic zone. A cross sectional, retrospective study in 45 subjects with 2 to 4 year follow up. J Periodontol. 2008;79:1773–81.
2. Hammerle CH, Lang NP. Single stage surgery combining transmucosal implant placement with guided bone regeneration and bioresorbable materials. Clin Oral Implants Res. 2001;12:9–18.
3. Hurzeler MB, Strub JR. Guided bone regeneration around exposed implants. A new bioresorbable device and bioresorbable membrane pins. Pract Periodontics Aesthet Dent. 1995;7:37–47.
4. Buser D, Dahlin C. Bone grafts and bone substitute materials. In: Buser D, editor. Guided bone regeneration in implant dentistry. 2nd ed. Chicago, IL: Quintessence; 2009. p. 71–96.
5. Dahlin C, Linde A, Gottlow J, Nyman S. Healing of bone defects by guided tissue regeneration. Plast Reconstr Surg. 1988;81:672–6.
6. Gottlow J. Guided tissue regeneration using bioresorbable and non resorbable devices. Initial healing and long term results. J Periodontol. 1993;64:1157–65.
7. Neukam FW, Mosgau SS. Implantate bei ausgedehnten Knochendefiziten. In: Koeck B, Wagner W, editors. Implantologie. Wrocław: Urban i Partner; 2004. p. 200–15.
8. Buser D, Dula K, Belser U, Hirt HP, Berthold H. Localized ridge augmentation using guided bone regeneration. 2. Surgical procedure in the mandible. Int J Periodontics Restorative Dent. 1995;15:10–29.
9. Urban IA, Lozada JL, Jovanovic SA, Nagursky H, Nagy K. Vertical ridge augmentation with titanium reinforced membranes and a combination of particulated autogenous bone and anorganic bovine bone derived mineral: a prospective case series in 19 patients. Int J Oral Maxillofac Implants. 2014;29:185–93.
10. Von Arz T, Buser D. Horizontal ridge augmentation using autogenous block grafts and the guided bone regeneration technique with collagen membranes: a clinical study with 42 patients. Clin Oral Implants Res. 2006;17:359–66.

11. Nentwig GH. Technic of bone splitting for alveolar recession in anterior maxillary region. Quintessenz. 1986;37:1825–34.
12. Hölzle F, Bauer F, Kesting MR, Mücke T, Deppe H, Wolff KD, Swaid S. Single stage implantation in the atrophy alveolar ridge of the mandible with the Norian skeletal repair system. B J Oral Maxillofac Surg. 2011;49(7):542–5.

Sinus Augmentation

4

Eric Kok Weng Lye and Winston Kwong Shen Tan

4.1 Definition

Maxillary sinus lift (also known as sinus grafting, sinus augmentation or sinus procedure) is a surgical procedure to increase the amount of alveolar bone in the maxilla (upper jaw bone), commonly in the area of the premolar and molar teeth, by lifting the Schneiderian membrane (sinus membrane) of the maxillary sinus floor and placing the graft material in the space.

The objective of the procedure is to correct deficient bone foundation in order to support dental implants in the posterior maxillary alveolar ridge. The adequacy of alveolar bone in the posterior maxilla is dependent on three factors, the pneumatisation of the maxillary sinus (see Sect. 4.3) and the alveolar bone remodelling after loss of teeth and the degree of alveolar bone development for congenitally missing teeth.

E. K. W. Lye (✉)
The Oral Maxillofacial Practice, Singapore, Singapore

Division of Oral and Maxillofacial Surgery, Ng Teng Fong General Hospital, Singapore, Singapore

Department of Otorhinolaryngology, Changi General Hospital, Singapore, Singapore

Department of Oral and Maxillofacial Surgery and OSA Clinic, National Dental Centre, Singapore, Singapore
e-mail: admin@omfp.com.sg

W. K. S. Tan
The Oral Maxillofacial Practice, Singapore, Singapore

Division of Oral and Maxillofacial Surgery, Ng Teng Fong General Hospital, Singapore, Singapore
e-mail: winston@omfp.com.sg

A. S. Budihardja, T. Mücke (eds.), *Bone Management in Dental Implantology*,
https://doi.org/10.1007/978-3-319-78951-4_4

When a tooth is lost, the tooth socket starts to heal leaving an edentulous (toothless) area. This process is known as remodelling and causes a variable loss in both height and width of the surrounding bone. The amount of shrinkage during remodelling is influenced by periodontal disease and trauma from the extraction procedure. The maxillary sinus also undergoes pneumatisation after extraction, causing the sinus floor to expand inferiorly at the extraction site [1]. As a result, this may lead to insufficient bone mass for osseointegration of titanium implant fixtures.

4.2 History

In 1960, Dr. Philip Boyne suggested lifting the maxillary sinus floor in order to increase vertical inter-ridge space for denture fabrication [2]. Subsequently in 1974, Dr. Hilt Tatum Jr. performed the first maxillary sinus lift augmentation procedure to aid in dental endosseous implant treatment. It was successful and allowed the subsequent placement of two endosseous implants [3].

4.2.1 Lateral Window Technique

The procedure was initially performed using inflatable catheters before specific sinus lift instruments were designed. The first technique used by Tatum involved opening a bony window in the lateral wall of the sinus. An autogenous bone was then placed in the space created by lifting the sinus membrane from the floor. This was the basis of the lateral window technique.

4.2.2 Crestal Approach

It was only in 1994 that Dr. Summers proposed the crestal or transcrestal approach, with placement of the graft from the implant osteotomy sites. This technique eliminated the need for the additional opening to the sinus via the lateral window [4].

4.3 Anatomy

The maxillary sinus is one of the four paired paranasal sinuses in the human skull. They are named according to the bones they are located in. These are the maxillary, ethmoid, frontal and sphenoidal sinuses. Paranasal sinuses are initially formed prenatally as small air-filled cavities that progressively erode into the bones surrounding the nasal cavity. They continue growing in size through life. The formed sinus cavities are connected to the nasal cavity through small openings called ostia.

4.3.1 Boundaries

The maxillary sinus is found in the body of the maxillary bone (Fig. 4.1). Its shape is similar to a pyramid with the base being the anterior maxillary wall. The superior wall is the floor of the orbit. The posterolateral wall is made of the zygomatic bone and greater wing of the sphenoid bone. Its medial wall is the lateral nasal wall composed of the inferior nasal concha, the palatine bone, the uncinate process of the ethmoid bone and the lacrimal bone. The inferior wall (sinus floor) sits above the alveolar bone of the posterior maxilla and is formed by the lateral nasal bone and the anterior sinus wall. This results in a cavity of mean volume of 10 ml.

4.3.2 Functional Drainage

The ostium of maxillary sinus is located two-thirds up the lateral nasal wall, draining into the middle meatus, exiting the lower portion of the hiatus semilunaris (Fig. 4.2). It is approximately 2.4 mm in diameter.

Sinus cavities are lined by a respiratory lining (pseudostratified columnar epithelium). In the maxillary sinus, this is also known as the "Schneiderian membrane". From endoscopic biopsies, the mean thickness of healthy sinus membranes is 0.97 mm [5]. This is close to the 0.8 ± 1.2 mm thickness measured using computed tomography (CT) [6]. The lining cells have cilia projections that help to sweep the contents of the cavities through the ostia into the nasal cavity. This mechanism is

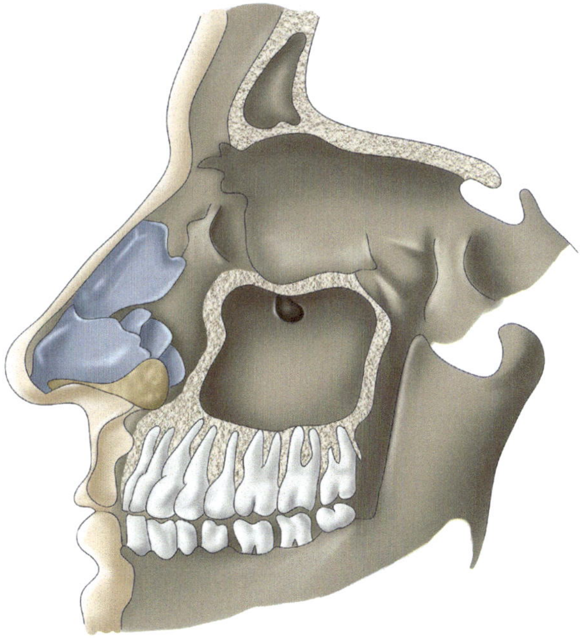

Fig. 4.1 Lateral view of the bones of the face with a portion of the zygomatic bone removed to show the maxillary alveolus and its relationship with the bony boundaries of the maxillary sinus. Of note is the superiorly positioned drainage point of the sinus (ostium)

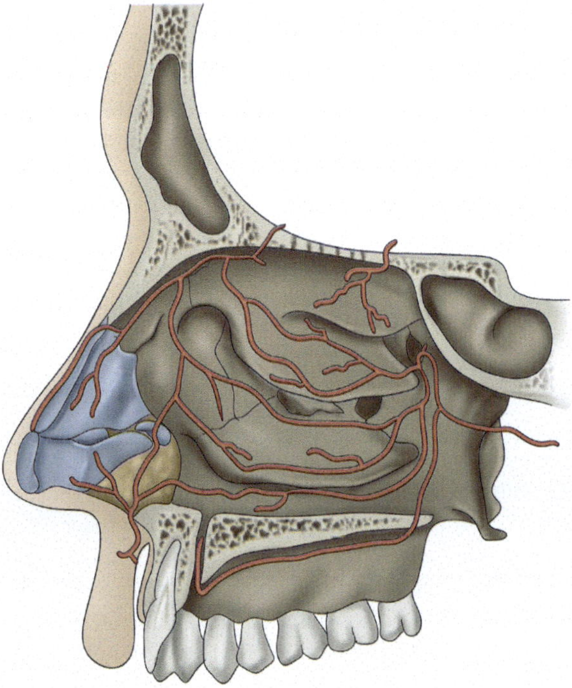

Fig. 4.2 Medial view of the maxillary sinus showing thc position of the ostium draining into middle meatus, at the lower portion of the hiatus semilunaris. It also illustrates its rich blood supply from the anterior ethmoidal, posterior ethmoidal, sphenopalatine and descending palatine arteries

especially important for the maxillary sinus as its ostium is found at the upper medial corner of the cavity and its drainage cannot be aided by gravity. If the drainage of the sinus is defective or obstructed, mucous secretions accumulate in the sinus cavities and may lead to sinus infection.

4.3.3 Blood Supply

The sinus has a rich blood supply. It is vascularised from the ethmoidal arteries (anterior and posterior), the sphenopalatine and descending palatine arteries (Fig. 4.2). There is also supply to the lateral wall and floor from the infraorbital, greater palatine and posterior superior alveolar arteries. Of surgical significance is the anastomosis between the posterior superior and infraorbital artery (Fig. 4.3). It consists of an extra- and intraosseous component. The extraosseous anastomosis is inconsistent and presents approximately only a third of the time [7]. The constant intraosseous portion is found from 16 to 19 mm superior to the alveolar crest [8]. Significant intraoperative bleeding may be encountered when it is traumatised during surgery.

4.4 Indications and Contraindications for Sinus Augmentation

Sinus augmentation (sinus lift) is performed when there is insufficient vertical bone height at the area of the maxilla where dental implants are to be placed. This procedure is performed to ensure an adequate bone foundation for the implants while

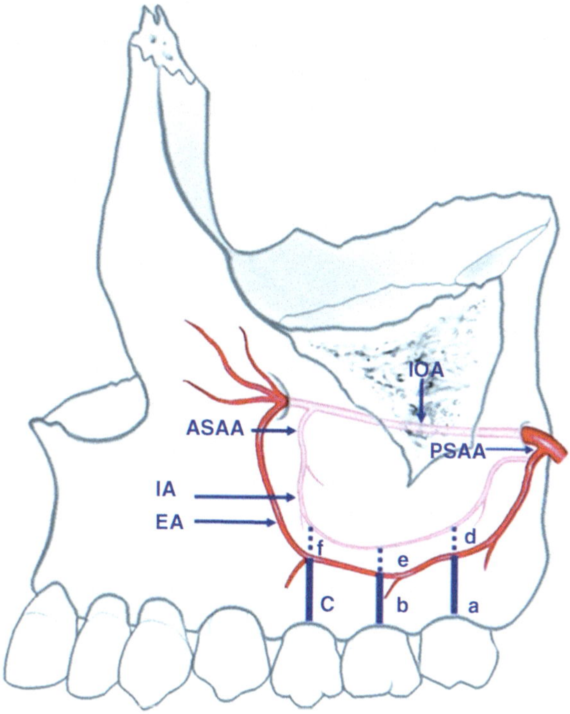

Fig. 4.3 View of the lateral maxillary sinus wall, showing the intraosseous and extraosseous anastomoses between the infraorbital and posterior superior alveolar arteries. The intraosseous anastomosis is a consistent vessel within the lateral wall of the sinus with mean distances to the alveolar ridge of 17.7 mm for the second maxillary molar, 14.5 mm for the first maxillary molar and 14.7 mm for the second maxillary premolar [36]

protecting the sinus (Fig. 4.4). As a rule of thumb, the bone should be augmented to accommodate an implant of at least 10 mm in height.

4.4.1 Indications

Patients who have the following may be good candidates for sinus augmentation:

- One or more missing teeth in the posterior maxilla secondary to loss or agenesis.
- Less than 8 mm of vertical alveolar bone height in the posterior maxilla.

4.4.2 Contraindications

- Active maxillary sinusitis (Fig. 4.5) is a contraindication for sinus lifting. It has to be resolved prior to graft placement.
- Active and chronic periodontitis are associated with increased sinus graft infection and implant failure [9].

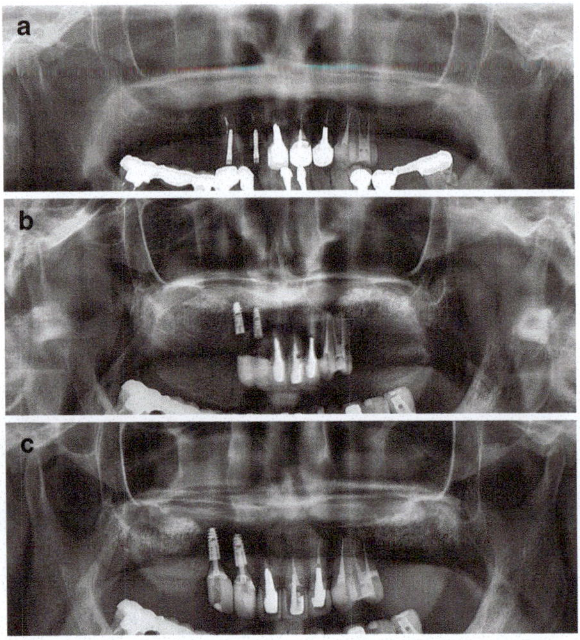

Fig. 4.4 (**a**) Presurgical panoramic view showing insufficient bone in the posterior maxilla for implant placement. (**b**) Immediate postsurgical panoramic view showing addition of bovine xenograft bilaterally and concurrent implant placement in the right maxilla. (**c**) Six-month postsurgical panoramic view showing mature bovine xenograft bilaterally and restored right maxillary implants. Please note that at this timeline the xenograft is not fully replaced with new bone growth, but is stable enough to support the placement of dental implants

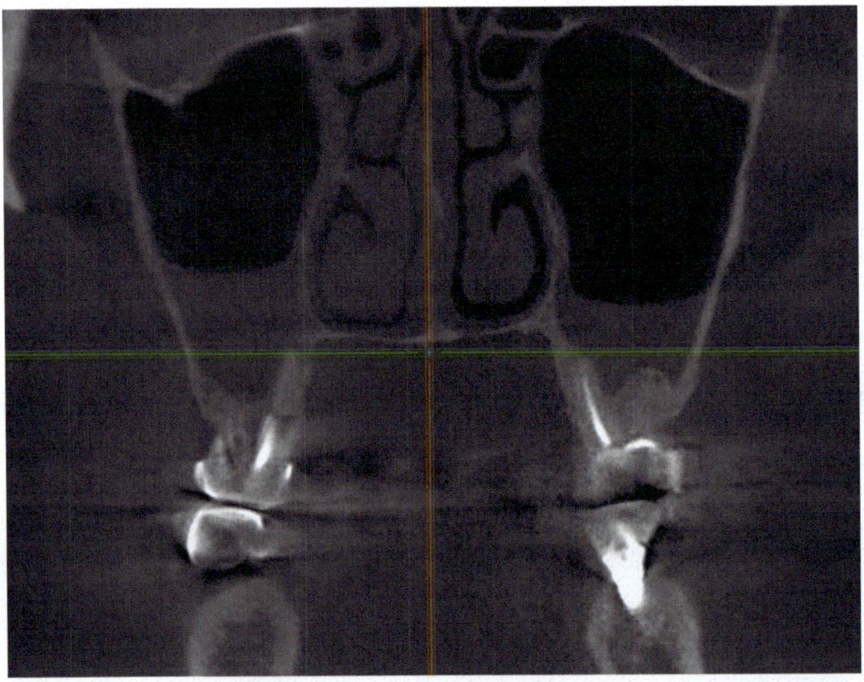

Fig. 4.5 Cone beam CT scan showing bilateral maxillary sinusitis with fluid levels

- Oro-antral communication (perforations and fistulas) at implant site.
- Heavy smokers are a relative contraindication and should be counselled on the increased risk of implant and graft failure [10].
- Antral cysts and thickening of the Schneiderian membrane make the sinus lift (Fig. 4.6) technically harder and are also relative risks.

4.5 Sinus Lift Techniques

There are two basic methods for performing the sinus lift technique (Fig. 4.7). These are the lateral window and crestal approach techniques.

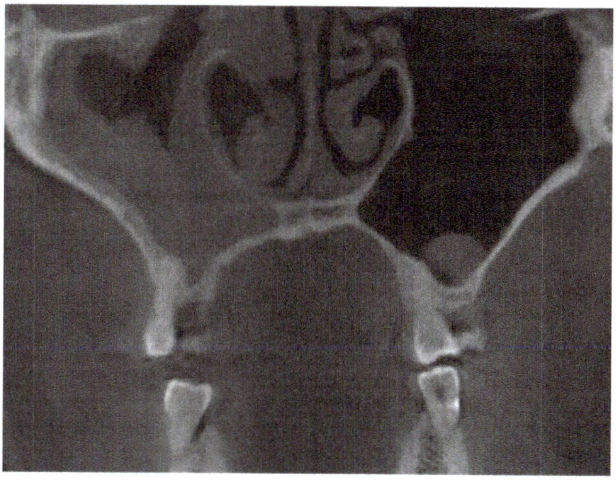

Fig. 4.6 Cone beam CT scan showing extensive thickening of the right maxillary sinus. The left maxillary sinus shows presence of an antral cyst. The presence of sinus pathology makes the sinus lift technically more difficult and at higher risk for developing complications

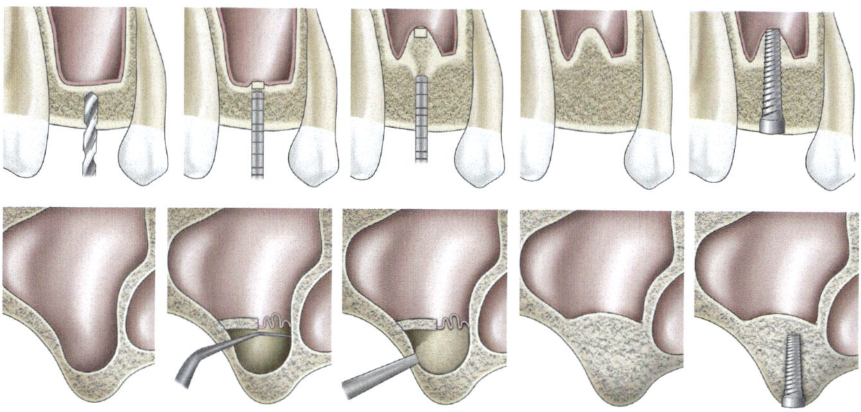

Fig. 4.7 Different techniques for sinus augmentation. The crestal technique (top) relies on osteotomes to raise the bony floor from the implant preparation sites and often involved simultaneous placement of dental implants. The lateral window technique (bottom) involved making a lateral osteotomy and lifting the sinus membrane with instruments placed on from the buccal side. Depending on the existing quality of the sinus floor, implants may be also placed (but less commonly) at the same time of the augmentation

4.5.1 Lateral Window Technique

Since 1974, the lateral window approach has been the workhorse for sinus augmentation. Opening a window in the lateral wall of the sinus allows for direct visualisation of the bone defect and sinus lining. It also allows for a larger volume graft to be placed in the sinus. However, it is a more invasive procedure, with increased morbidity, such as swelling, bruising and pain. This technique is valuable in augmentation of severely resorbed sites (Fig. 4.7).

4.5.2 Crestal Approach

In 1994, Summers, who was in pursuit of a less invasive sinus lift method, made the surgical protocol easier by offering a crestal approach or osteotome technique [4]. Initially, osteotomes were used for condensing the soft maxillary bone surrounding implant osteotomy sites. This was to improve the initial stability and success rates of implants placed in the posterior maxilla. After a period of success using this technique for bone compression, Summers started floor dilatation of the sinus, thus increasing the length of his implants. Osteotomes were used to infracture the sinus floor. Bone graft material was then inserted from the crest, lifting the lining in the process (Fig. 4.7).

There were two disadvantages with the crestal approach. The first disadvantage was the limited amount of vertical augmentation achievable. Summers was able to lift the membrane 1–3 mm only. The second limitation was the inability to directly visualise the membrane.

Generally, the more conservative crestal technique is recommended when 4–6 mm of residual bone height is present, and an increase of 3–5 mm of bone can be realistically achieved for an 8 mm implant. When more advanced resorption is present, the lateral window technique should be performed. When performed without complications, both techniques would not affect the implant success rate [11].

It takes about 3–6 months for the sinus augmentation bone to become part of the patient's natural sinus floor bone. Sometimes healing of up to 9 months may be necessary before implant insertion is attempted [12]. It is possible to avoid the necessity of two surgeries if implants can be successfully placed with the sinus augmentation [13].

4.6 Presurgical Evaluation

4.6.1 Radiographic Evaluation

Panoramic radiographs can be used to assess the vertical dimension of the maxillary alveolus but are sometimes inadequate to diagnose sinus disease or variations like intraosseous arteries and sinus septa (Fig. 4.8a, b). If there are suspicions of abnormalities, a computed tomography or CT scan is taken to determine the sinus' exact height and width and to rule out any sinus disease or pathology [14].

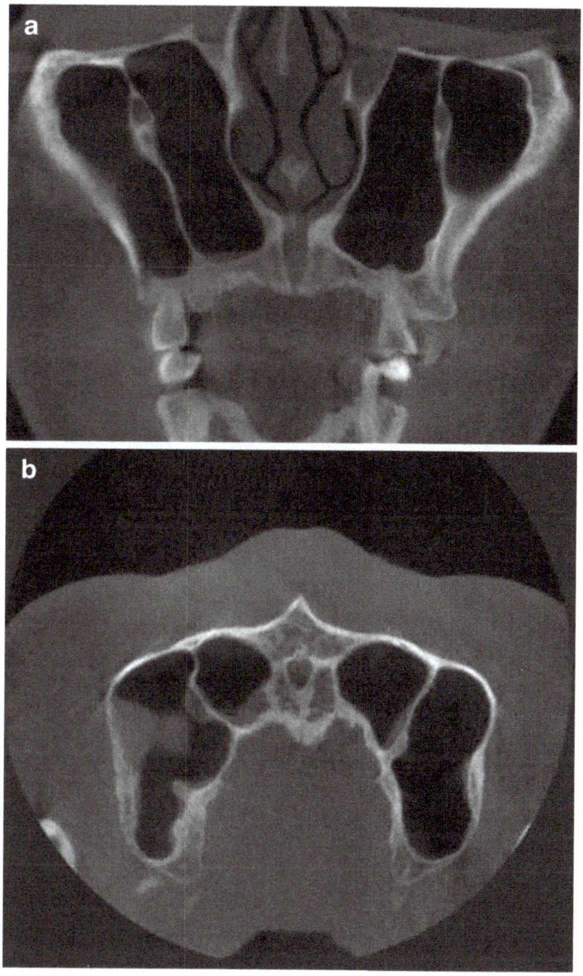

Fig. 4.8 (**a**) Coronal view of a cone beam CT scan showing the anatomy of the sinus septa. The location of the septa may influence the augmentation technique used. (**b**) Axial view of a cone beam CT scan showing the sinus septa. The location of the septa may influence the augmentation technique used (both scans are of the same patient). Please also note the narrow cross section at the anterior maxilla compared to the posterior region

The thickness of the lateral wall of the maxillary sinus can be evaluated from a CT scan. It ranges from 0.5 to 2.5 mm [15]. Very thin or very thick sinus walls may complicate the lateral window technique.

The bony septa within the sinus in the site of the augmentation may complicate the procedure and dictate the technique to be used. For example, vertical septa in the area where an implant needs to be placed may prevent the clinician from carrying out the osteotome technique (Fig. 4.9).

4.6.2 Alveolar Ridge Morphology

The pre-existing alveolar bone width in the bucco-palatal dimension is also an important determinant in the decision-making process. A thin bone may require grafting in the horizontal dimension with block or particulate grafts in addition to vertical augmentation via the sinus lift. In the case of patients with irregular ridge

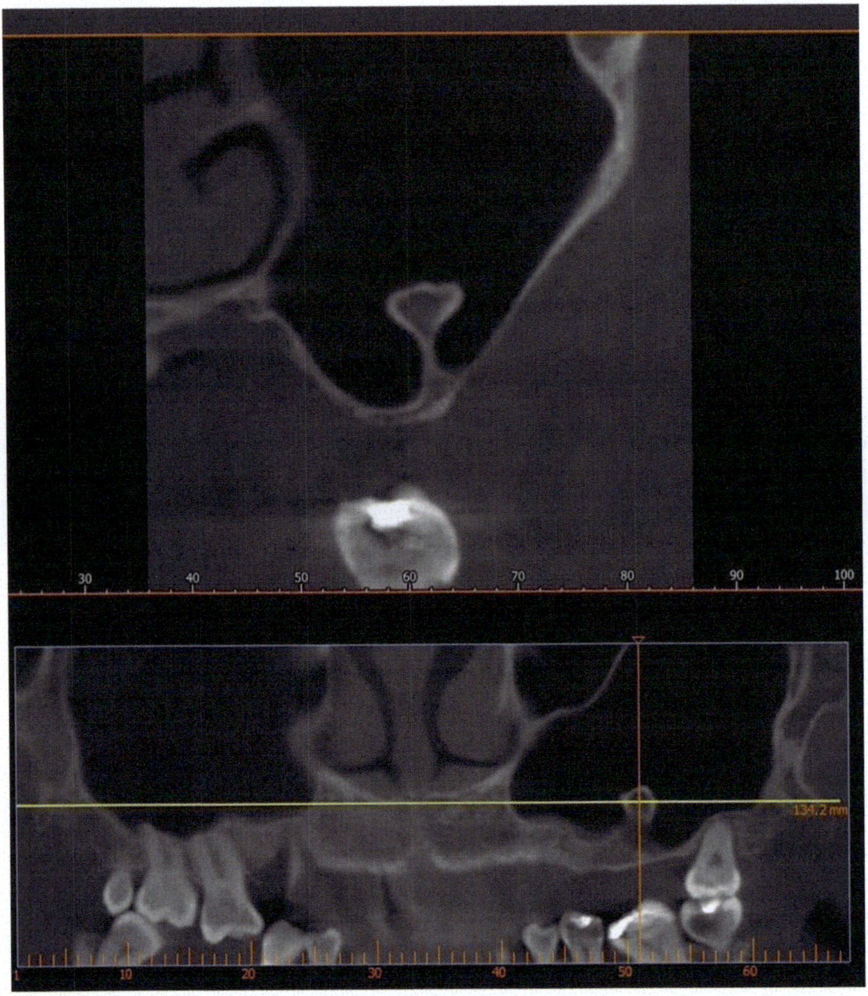

Fig. 4.9 Panoramic and cross-sectional view of the left maxillary sinus as seen on cone beam CT scan. The presence of the heart-shaped septa at the upper left molar area makes a crestal approach very difficult

morphology, calculations should also be made to compensate for any concurrent alveolar reduction.

4.7 Lateral Window Technique

4.7.1 Lateral Window Technique: Surgery

4.7.1.1 Radiographic Examination

This is made with a panoramic radiograph and a cone beam CT where deemed necessary (Fig. 4.10). Occasionally, superimposition of other anatomical structures in

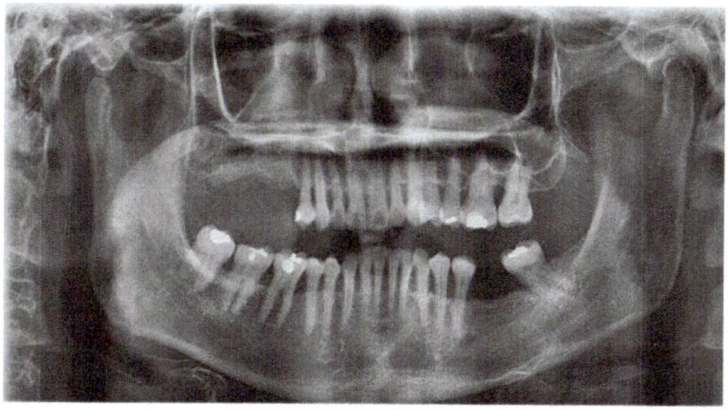

Fig. 4.10 Presurgical panoramic radiograph showing an edentulous span in the upper right maxilla for sinus lift surgery and implant placement. Clinical photographs in Fig. 4.11 are of the same patient

the panoramic view can prevent accurate visualisation of the sinus floor, and a confirmatory CT will aid in accurate diagnosis.

4.7.1.2 Incision

A mucoperiosteal gingival flap is raised using a crestal incision with vertical relieving incisions. The authors recommend an incision over the crest of the ridge with a band of attached mucosa. This is usually mid-crestal to a slightly palatal position (Fig. 4.11a, b). The vertical incisions should be placed so that they lie over the sound bone at closure. In some cases, it means the incisions are placed one tooth anterior and posterior beyond the lateral window. The length of the vertical release should allow adequate exposure of the lateral bony wall of the sinus.

4.7.1.3 Lateral Window Osteotomy

The boundaries of the sinus cavity can usually be visualised by an increase in translucency of the overlying bone. The lateral window osteotomy is made over the translucent areas, and its dimensions are determined by the following parameters (Fig. 4.11c, d):

- Inferior horizontal cut should be placed 1–2 mm above the (measured) sinus floor. This allows for containment of the graft material. At the same time, it allows for the working end of sinus lift instruments to reach the floor, reducing the risk of tearing of the fragile membrane.
- Superior horizontal cut should be placed at the upper limit of the planned implant height. For example, if a 10 mm implant is to be placed in the site, the authors recommend the superior horizontal cut be placed 10–12 mm from the crest of the ridge.
- Anterior vertical cut should follow the sloping anterior floor of the sinus and be placed 1–2 mm anterior to the planned grafting site to allow for easy access and to reduce the risk of tearing of the membrane. The anterior portion of the maxillary sinus is narrower in cross section compared to the rest of the sinus (Fig. 4.8b), and this increases the chance of a membrane perforation during elevation.
- Posterior vertical cut should be in line with the distal portion of the planned implant placement. This is less critical than the placement of the other cuts. The sinus lift instruments are manipulated from the front, so access to the posterior wall is less challenging.

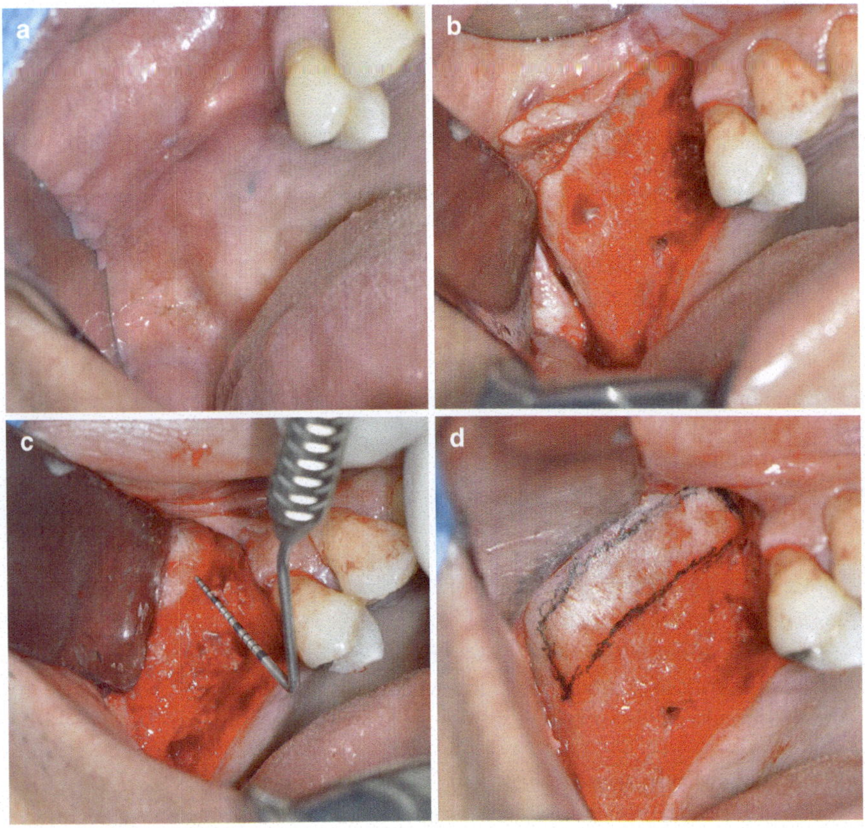

Fig. 4.11 (**a**, **b**) Exposure of the posterior maxilla via a crestal incision with vertical release incisions. The exposure should be planned so that the edges of the flap can rest on sound bone. (**c**, **d**) Defining the bony margins of the lateral window osteotomy. Measurements may be made with a periodontal probe, and the margins can be outlined with a surgical pencil (Sect. 4.7.1.3). (**e**, **f**) The bone cuts of the lateral window osteotomy can be made with a standard 2 mm diameter surgical round bur (**e**), or a piezotome (**f**) may be used. (**g**, **h**) The outline of the bony window prior to lifting the sinus membrane (**g**). This window may be preserved and infractured or carefully removed to expose the sinus membrane (**h**). (**i**, **j**) Elevating the sinus membrane from the lateral window osteotomy. In this example, the bony window is teased away from the membrane and removed. The translucent sinus membrane is now completely exposed. If intact, it will move in sync with the patient's respiration. (**k**, **l**) Elevating the sinus membrane from the sinus floor. It is important to develop the lift from both the floor and the anterior vertical portion of the osteotomy. The sinus is narrower in the anterior and has in increased chance of tearing. (**m**, **n**) Repairing a membrane tear with bio-resorbable porcine collagen membrane. Small perforations can be repaired and the lift does not need to be abandoned. Elevating the membrane also reduces the size of the tear. (**o**) Preparing the implant sites for simultaneous implant placement. Care is taken to avoid perforation of the membrane during implant site preparation. (**p**, **q**) Bone is packed in the medial aspect of the sinus prior to implant insertion to ensure there is bone all around the implant surface. (**r**–**t**) The bone is packed on the lateral aspect of the implants. In this example, the harvested bony buccal window is replaced over the lateral surface prior to coverage with a bioresorbable porcine collagen membrane. (**u**) A watertight seal is made with interrupted sutures to close the wound. It is important that the flap rests on the sound bone and is not perforated. There is primary closure over the implants in this example, although it is possible to place healing abutments and carry out a single-stage surgery

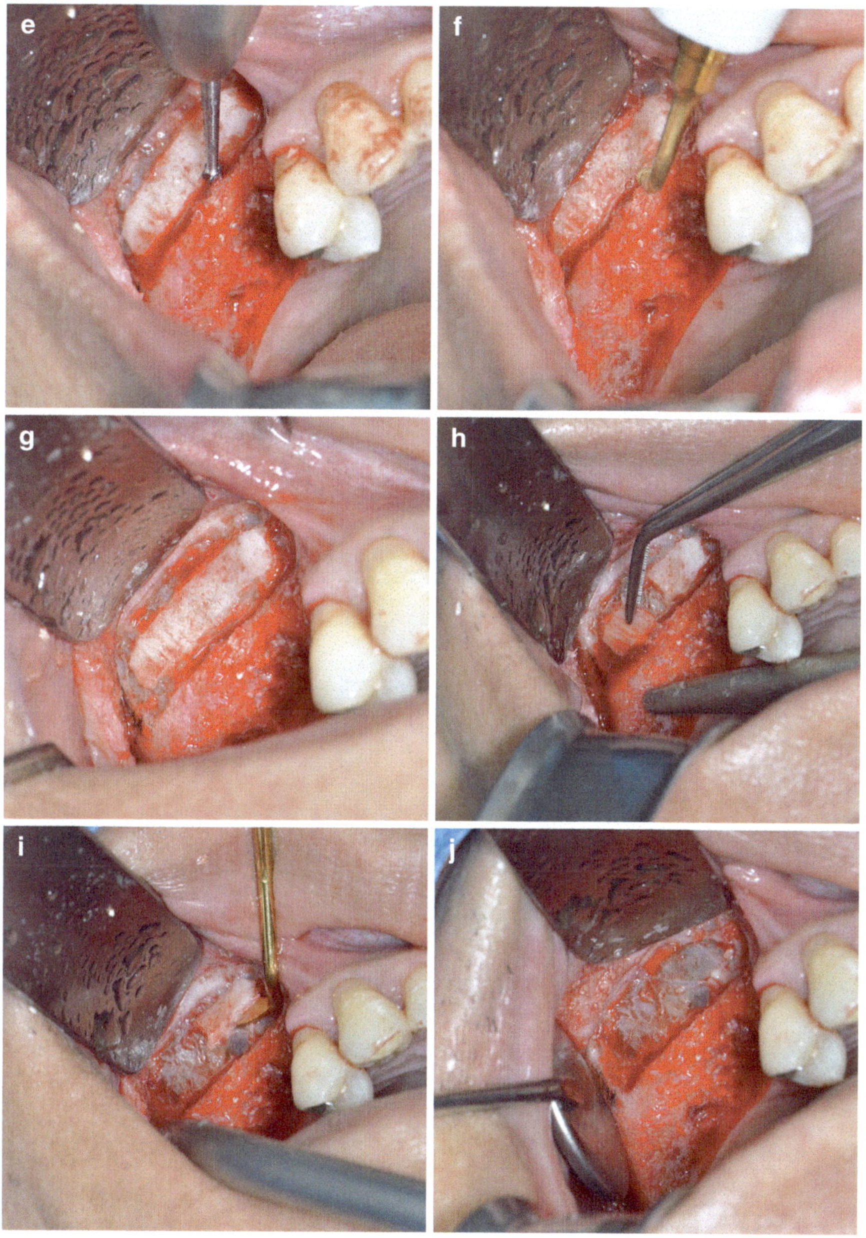

Fig. 4.11 (continued)

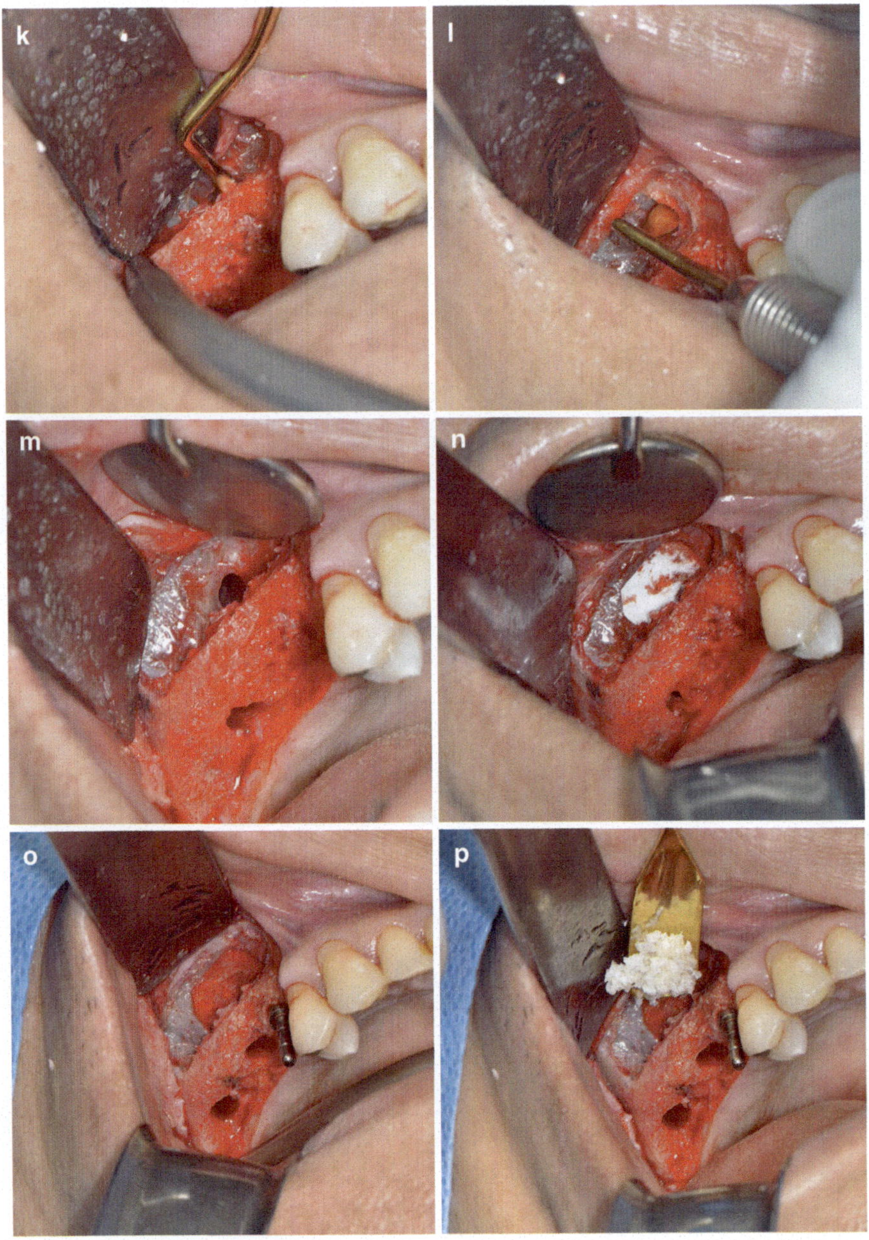

Fig. 4.11 (continued)

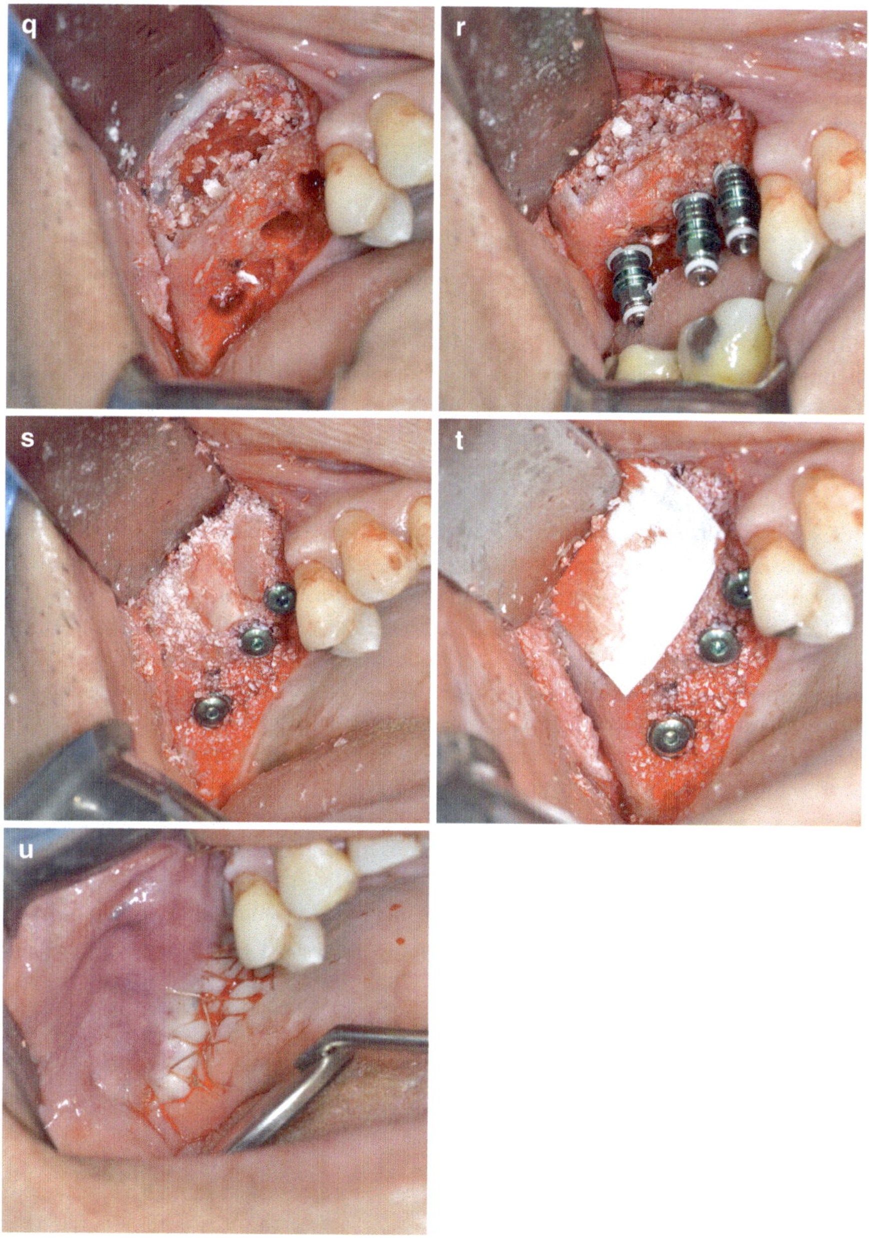

Fig. 4.11 (continued)

There are several methods to create the "window". Some surgeons will use a round diamond bur or a piezotome instead of a regular surgical bur (Fig. 4.11e, f) to reduce the potential for trauma to the underlying sinus lining [16]. The bony fragment in the "window" can be infractured and preserved or removed completely (Fig. 4.11g, h). These variations are not critical to the outcome of the lift and are based on personal preferences of the surgeon.

4.7.1.4 Sinus Elevation and Initial Graft Placement

The sinus membrane is then gently elevated from the inner wall of the antral cavity around the window and from the sinus floor (Fig. 4.11i, l). An intact membrane (Fig. 4.11j) will move according to the breathing of the patient. Although an intact membrane is best, perforation of the membrane does not mean the lift needs to be abandoned (Fig. 4.11m, n). Subsequently, bone graft material is placed into the newly created space and packed on the medial surface. This creates a border of bone on the medial side of any implants that are placed simultaneously.

4.7.1.5 Simultaneous Implant Placement

It is possible to place implants together with the lateral window technique if there is enough bone present for primary implant stability. If an implant is placed simultaneously with the lateral window technique, bone is inserted to the palatal portion of the space created prior to implant placement to ensure there is a bone on both the medial and lateral surfaces of the implant (Fig. 4.11o, q). Another useful trick is to also insert bone via the implant osteotomy and condensing it, as one would do with the crestal technique. This ensures that the bone is packed all around the periphery of the implant.

In cases of simultaneous implant placement, the clinician should be mindful that the posterior maxillary bone is soft and porous. The use of condensing osteotomes and the under-preparation of the implant sites are useful tricks to increase the primary stability when implants are inserted. However, care must be taken not to fracture the remaining thin lateral wall when this is carried out. This will result in significant bone loss due to the inability to confine the graft in the native bone.

4.7.1.6 Lateral Surface of the Bone Graft

The lateral wall is usually covered with a barrier membrane to prevent fibrous ingrowth from the mucosa and gingiva [17]. The authors commonly use resorbable porcine collagen membrane for this purpose. The use of a barrier membrane, however, is debatable with some suggesting that it does not change the implant survival rate [18, 19].

4.7.1.7 Wound Closure

As mentioned earlier, it is good practice to raise a flap that is one tooth broader than the lateral window to be created. This allows for it to be replaced on sound bone after the graft has been added. The flap is then sutured, and the graft is left to heal for 4–9 months, depending on the material used and the volume of augmentation beyond the native bone (Fig. 4.11u) [12]. If implants have been placed and there is

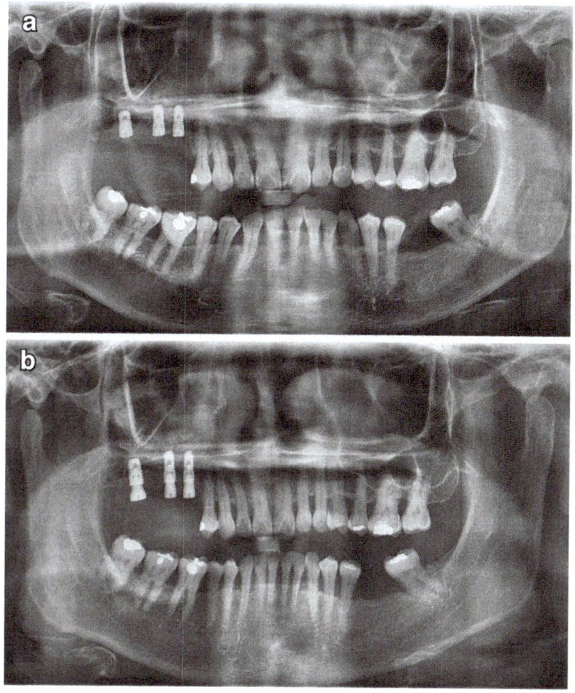

Fig. 4.12 (a) Immediate postoperative panoramic view of the lateral window lift with simultaneous implant placement (steps in Fig. 4.11). (b) Postoperative panoramic view of the lateral window lift at stage II surgery with placement of healing abutments (steps in Fig. 4.11). Note the changes in radiographic appearance of the graft material during the consolidation process

good confidence that the sinus has not been breached, it is possible to place healing abutments and treat this as a single-stage surgery. However, if in doubt, then primary closure of the wound is recommended.

The integrity of the mucoperiosteal flap is paramount in success of the lateral window sinus lift. It is critical to preserve the integrity of the gingival flap overlying the graft material to avoid infection of the graft. If the gingival flap is torn, it is recommended that a fat pad be used to protect the graft.

The entire sequence for the lateral window technique is depicted in Fig. 4.11. The postoperative radiographs are shown in Fig. 4.12a, b. The procedure is illustrated in Fig. 4.13.

4.7.2 Lateral Window Technique: Technical Tips

4.7.2.1 Membrane Perforation

This is a fairly common occurrence with the lateral window lift. This can be prevented with the use of diamond burs or specially created piezotome tips for the bony osteotomy. The use of dedicated instruments to tease the sinus lining off the roof of the alveolus also reduces the chance of perforation. High-risk areas for perforation correspond to the narrow sloping anterior wall, the presence of septa and the roof above recent extraction and sites where tooth roots have made undulations in the sinus floor.

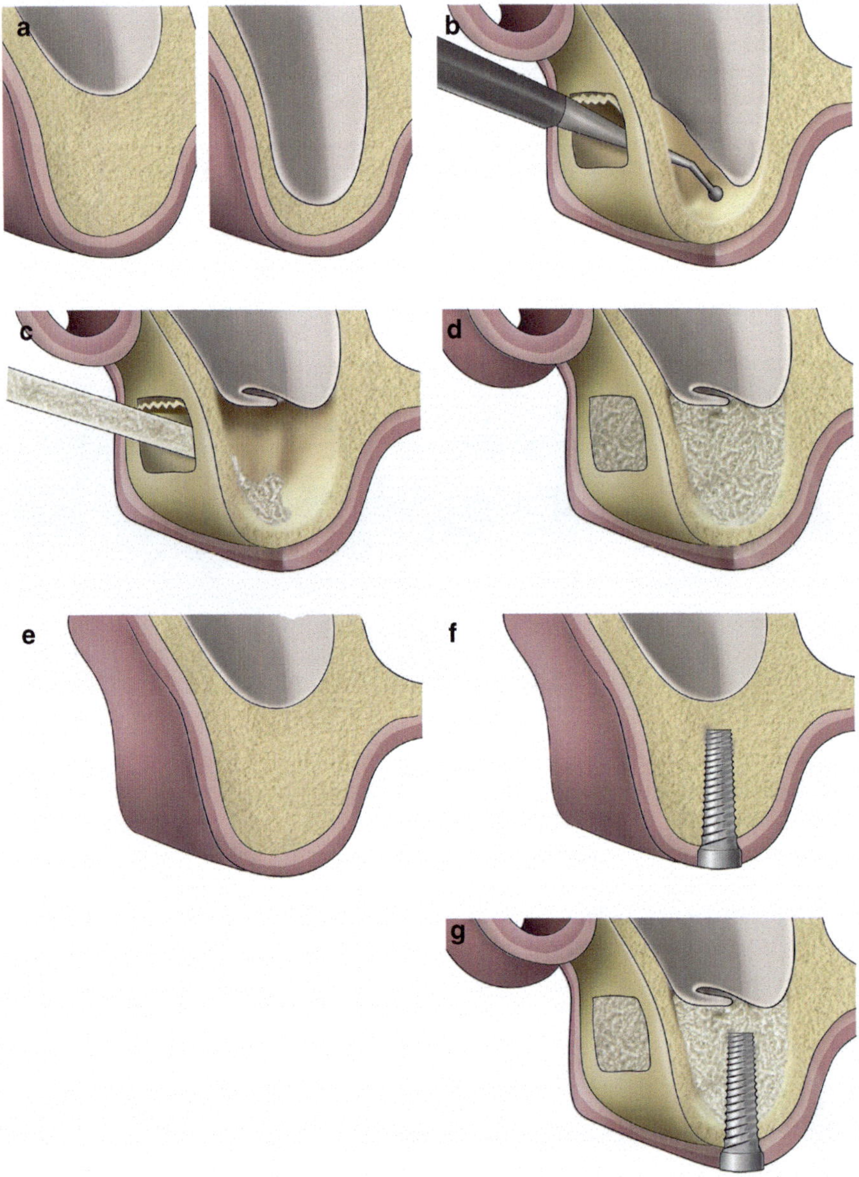

Fig. 4.13 Diagram illustrating the sequence of the lateral window sinus lift without and with simultaneous implant placement. Comparing the deficiency of the alveolar bone and planning the position of the lateral window (**a**). In sequence: opening of the bony window and lifting of the sinus lining (**b**), placement of the graft material (**c**), closure and bone maturity (**d**, **e**) and finally implant placement (**f**). Simultaneous implant placement requires the slight modification of packing of the graft on the medial surface prior to implant placement and the need to ensure implant stability (**g**)

The thickness of the sinus lining also has an impact on perforation with membrane with thicknesses of ≥3 and ≤0.5 mm having higher risk. Linings between 1 and 2 mm of thickness have the lowest risk [20].

When a perforation has occurred, the surgeon has to make a decision on whether to continue or abort the surgery. For small perforations of less than 5 mm in diameter, often the act of lifting the sinus lining off the floor can result in closure of the perforation, due to the geometry of converting a curved arc into a straight line (Fig. 4.13c). A membrane may also be inserted to seal off the tear (Fig. 4.11m, n), and a sign of achieving a successful seal is the moving of the membrane in sync with the patient's respiration. For large perforations, the objective is to prevent graft material from dispersing into the sinus. Tissue glue with a combination of large membranes may be effective in containing the material. When in doubt, the author's recommendation is to allow the membrane to heal (6–8 weeks) before reentering the site.

4.7.2.2 Narrow Lateral Window

Narrow sites of a single premolar width in the mesiodistal dimension are technically more challenging to carry out than wider edentulous spans, and the surgeon should be mindful of the increased difficulty and risk of membrane tear. A useful trick is to use a narrow, rounded instrument such as a plastic instrument for composite application to lift the membrane in confined spaces around the roots of the adjacent teeth.

4.8 Crestal (Osteotome or Transcrestal) Approach

4.8.1 Crestal (Osteotome or Transcrestal) Approach: Surgery

As an alternative, sinus augmentation can be performed by a less invasive osteotome technique. This is normally performed when the sinus floor needs to be lifted less than 5 mm (pre-existing subantral bone height of 4–6 mm) [21]. The amount of augmentation achieved with the crestal approach is less than what can be achieved with the lateral window technique. A dental implant is normally placed at the same sitting and left to integrate with the bone. Bone graft integration normally takes 4–9 months, depending on the amount of lifting carried out and the type of bone graft used [19]. The entire sequence of the crestal approach is depicted below (Fig. 4.14a–d).

4.8.1.1 Radiographic Examination

It is necessary to examine the radiograph (panoramic or cone beam CT) that the floor to be lifted has no septa (Fig. 4.9) or that it is not sloping. A sloping sinus floor presents a challenge for the internal lift, as one aspect is thin whilst the other side remains too thick for successful lifting. This slope also tends to drive the osteotome in the wrong direction (Fig. 4.15). In this situation, the clinician should consider the possibility of carrying out a lateral sinus lift in conjunction with implant placement for better control of the bone graft distribution and a lesser chance of violation of the integrity of the sinus membrane.

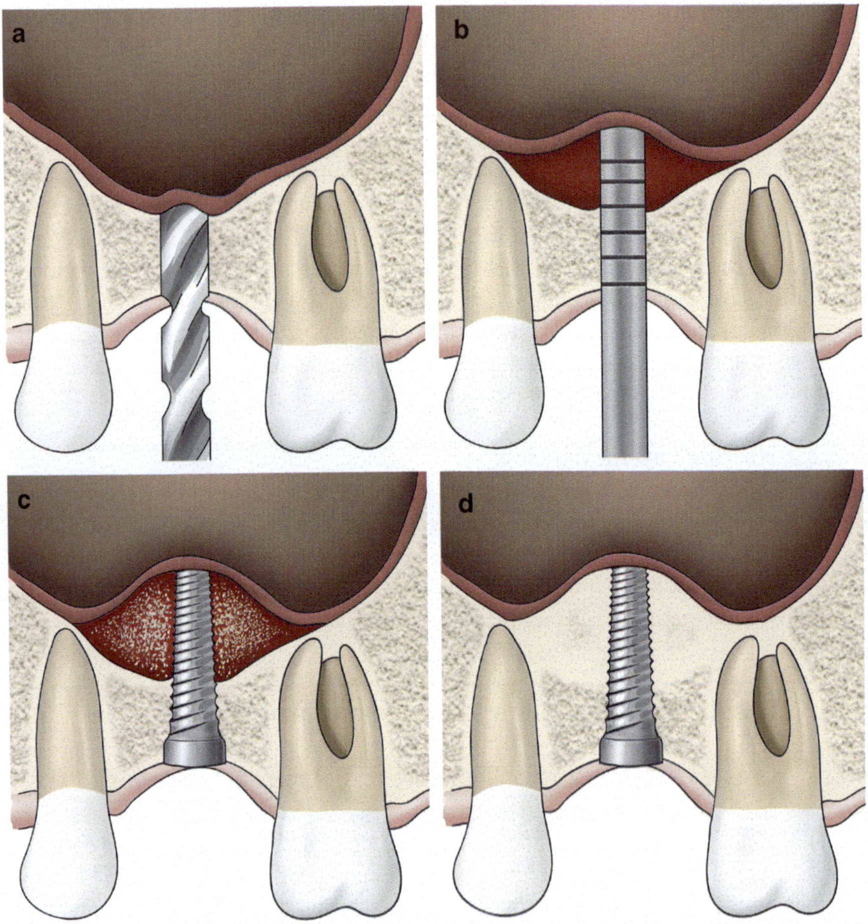

Fig. 4.14 (**a–d**) The sequence of the crestal approach using the sinus lift osteotome. Drilling is carried out to 1 mm short of the desired depth. The osteotome is inserted and the sinus floor and lining are lifted. Bone is packed and inserted via the implant site preparation. The implant is simultaneously inserted and the bone is allowed to mature

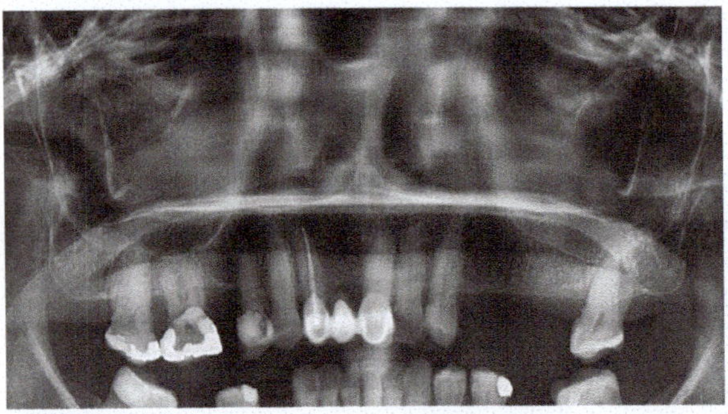

Fig. 4.15 Panoramic view of the maxilla. Note the sloping sinus floor in the upper left and right premolar regions, especially at the upper right second premolar area. Lifting of the sinus lining via the crestal approach needs to be done with care as the bone thickness is not uniform and the osteotome may be misdirected in the process

4.8.1.2 Incision

The crestal technique is performed by making an incision over the crest of the future implant site. In contrast to the lateral window technique, minimal releasing incisions need to be made. Incisions into the gingival sulcus of the adjacent teeth are usually sufficient for adequate surgical exposure. In a situation where there is no posterior tooth, as in the maxillary tuberosity region, a distobuccal release can be made into the attached mucosa to allow for reflection of the flap.

4.8.1.3 Crestal Osteotomy

A channel is made in the alveolar bone with sequential implant drills to the final implant diameter (usually 4–5 mm). The preparation should be made 1–2 mm short of the sinus floor. The sinus floor is then "lifted" by tapping it with the use of dedicated sinus lift osteotomes. These are specifically designed to lift the sinus floor as they have a circular cutting edge, resulting in a concave profile. A circular "disc" of bone is raised with the osteotome, and it in turn raises the sinus membrane without damaging it. Some sinus lift osteotomes are equipped with depth stoppers. This limits the height to which the osteotome may be inserted, so that the sinus membrane is not tensed or breached (Fig. 4.16).

4.8.1.4 Bone Graft Placement

Bone graft material is placed into the channel, and the osteotome is reinserted to depth to push the graft material superiorly, lifting the membrane off the floor.

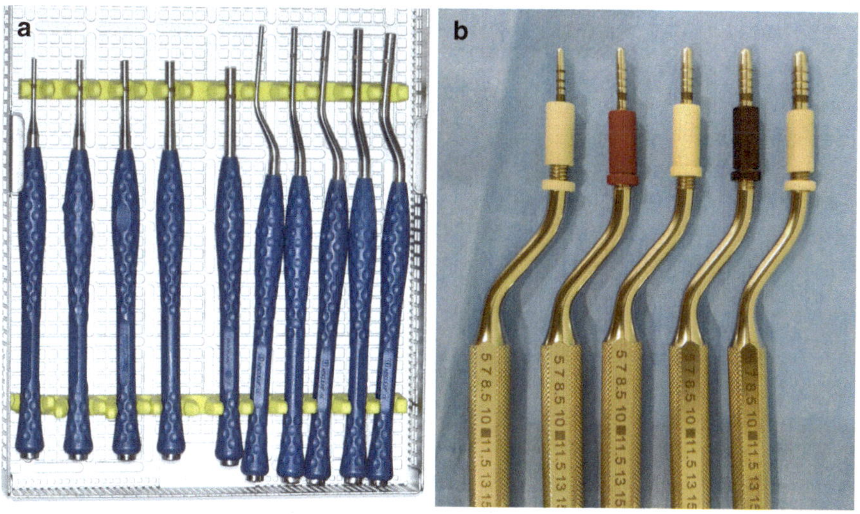

Fig. 4.16 (**a**) Sinus lift osteotomes. These are cylindrical in cross-section with a concave cutting tip. The osteotomes can also be fitted with depth stoppers to prevent unintentional intrusion into the sinus beyond the working length. (**b**) Condensing osteotomes. These are different from sinus lift osteotomes as they are intended to compress soft bone so as to increase the primary stability of the implant on insertion. They are not intended to cut at the working end, as so the tip of the osteotome is rounded

Specially designed carriers, which match the diameter of the osteotomy, may be used for this purpose. This process is repeated till the necessary volume of graft material has been placed into the site. It is important to note that the graft material is used to lift the membrane, rather than a direct application of the osteotome to the floor.

4.8.1.5 Implant Insertion and Wound Closure

The implant is then inserted, and a good primary stability must be achieved. The implant fixture should be placed slowly to allow the bone graft to settle around the apex and advance into the sinus. The site is then closed primarily over the implant with interrupted sutures. A healing abutment may be placed if the surgeon is confident of the initial stability of the implant and that the sinus lining has not been breached.

4.8.2 Crestal Approach: Technical Tips

4.8.2.1 Sinus Lift Kits

Special mention should be made of sinus lift kits for the crestal approach [22]. These have drills designed specifically for creating a circular osteotomy at the base of the sinus floor. They are touted to be less traumatic than conventional implant burs and are also available with depth stoppers to limit the risk of sinus tear (Fig. 4.17).

4.8.2.2 Membrane Perforation

Despite all the precautions, the membrane is often torn during the crestal procedure [23]. This can be repaired either with the insertion of a resorbable membrane via the osteotomy opening or a formal lateral window approach, and the membrane is repaired as described previously (Sect. 4.6.1).

4.8.2.3 Achieving Primary Stability

This tip applies to both the lateral window lift with simultaneous implant placement and the crestal approach. It may be difficult to achieve primary stability in the posterior maxilla due to the poor bone quality there. The authors recommend that the bone be assessed from the time the pilot drill is inserted. If there is a suspicion that the bone is soft, the drill is run slowly (under 200 RPM) and allowed to perforate the crestal cortical plate without tearing the sinus membrane. If the pilot drill can be easily inserted with minimal resistance, the recommendation is the use of condensing osteotomes (Fig. 4.16b) to widen the osteotomy site in order to compact the bone and to increase the potential for stability. Another approach is to stop one drill size narrower than the recommended diameter prior to implant insertion. With both these approaches, it is essential that the implant engages the cortical bone of the sinus floor and does not stop short and spin within the bone. The surgeon should be able to differentiate between the cortical bone (dense), alveolar bone (soft) and the sinus floor (dense). Running the bur at a slow speed (under 200 RPM) allows the clinician to appreciate these three layers.

Use range (Use ■)

USII	SSII	TSII	Ultra-wide	MS	OS
USIII	SSIII	TSIII			

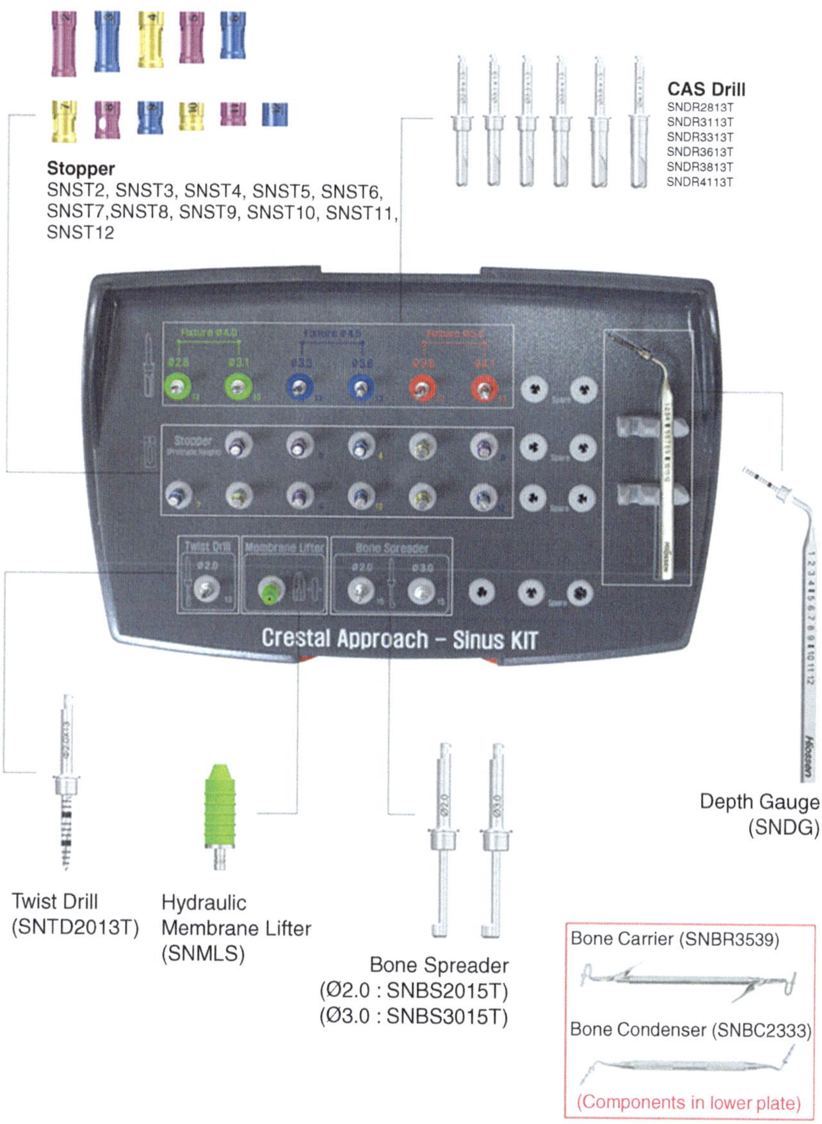

Fig. 4.17 Special kits designed for crestal approach sinus lifts. This example has specialised drills which are designed to minimise the perforation of the sinus membrane, as well as a hydraulic system to lift the membrane atraumatically. Special bone carriers are also included in this kit for placement of the graft material via the implant preparation site

4.9 Other Sinus Lift Techniques

4.9.1 Hydraulic Sinus Condensing Technique (HSC)

This technique was invented in 1996 by Dr. Leon Chen [24]. Other methods of lifting the sinus membrane are the Intralift™ from ACTEON [25], balloon sinus lifting [26] and sinus lifting with special burs that are also clinically proven [21, 27].

The HSC technique uses an osteotomy on the crestal aspect of the ridge of the maxilla. It has shown to have shorter recovery time than the traditional method. A dental implant is placed at the same time as the sinus lift, also reducing the time to fabrication of the final prosthesis.

A gingival flap is raised to access the underlying bone. An osteotomy (bone removal) is initiated along the ridge. Drilling ceases about 1 mm short of the sinus floor. Subsequently, a series of piezoelectric tips are used to widen and atraumatically puncture the sinus floor. Hydraulic pressure is then introduced to the surgical site at this stage, providing just enough force to begin dissecting the membrane from the sinus floor. Once the membrane is loosened, the hydraulic pressure is ceased. The membrane at rest is slightly detached from the bone. A bone grafting mixture is then packed through the hole and pushed gently against the membrane. This pressure teases up the sinus membrane, resting it on the newly placed bone.

Once the initial lift is complete, the surgeon creates an appropriate osteotomy in the bone that is sized to the new implant. Bone graft material is added again with pressure to further lift the sinus until it is raised to the proper height for implant placement. The surgeon then places the dental implant into the bone socket and sutures the gums back into place.

Over an 8-year study of 1557 implants in 1100 patients using the hydraulic sinus condensing technique, only eight implants failed, resulting in a 99.4% success rate [21].

4.10 Graft Materials Used in Sinus Augmentation

Autogenous bone. There are many different materials that can be used for sinus augmentation. The original material used was autogenous bone, which was then considered the gold standard [28].

Allografts are cadaveric bone that are harvested, processed and sterilised.

Xenografts are predominantly from bovine, porcine or equine sources with the organic components removed.

Alloplasts are synthetic bone substitutes with various chemical compositions such as beta-tricalcium phosphate, bioactive glass or calcium sulphate.

Studies suggest that a 50:50 mix of autogenous bone with the slow-resorbing xenograft bone yields the best balance between the transfer of active cellular components and long-term maintenance of the “space” for the new bone to grow.

The discovery of biologically active molecules, known as growth factors, led to their use. However, they also need an appropriate delivery system that will simulate natural bone formation [29].

Studies indicate that the mere lifting of the sinus membrane, creation of a void space and blood clot formation might result in a new bone owing to the principles of guided bone regeneration [30]. In some cases the dental implant is also inserted simultaneously during the sinus lift procedure. For all grafting techniques with simultaneous implant placement, primary stability is essential to prevent migration of the implant or implant and graft failure.

The research data comparing the various different materials in sinus augmentation did not show any significant advantages for any one of them [31].

4.11 Complications

4.11.1 Membrane Perforation

A major risk of a sinus augmentation is that the sinus membrane could be pierced or torn. The incidence of perforation is high and ranges from 20% to 44% in lateral approach and 0–25% in crestal approach [32]. Recommended remedies, should this occur, include stitching the tear or placing a membrane over it; in some cases, the surgery is aborted altogether, and the tear is given time to heal, usually for a minimum of 6–8 weeks (Sect. 4.8.2.2). It is the authors' experience that often the sinus membrane grows back thicker and stronger, making success more likely on the second operation.

A sinus perforation via the crestal approach may occasionally be repaired using the lateral window technique to go around the tear and repair it with the application of a membrane. In the situation where the surgeon feels that the tear cannot be repaired and would like to discontinue the surgery, it is recommended to apply a bioresorbable membrane to the lateral wall before closure. The resulting scar tissue has to be carefully dissected on reentry to prevent a new perforation and yet to maintain enough robustness in the buccal flap for a watertight final closure.

4.11.2 Maxillary Sinusitis

Besides tearing of the sinus membrane, there are other risks involved in sinus augmentation surgery. Most notably, the close relationship of the augmentation site with the sinonasal complex can induce sinusitis, which may become chronic and cause severe symptoms. In the preoperative assessment, patients with a history of sinus disease and sinus pathology should be appropriately counselled [3]. Patients with a higher risk of post-surgery blockage of the maxillary ostium (e.g. a deviated nasal septum) should also be counselled on their risks prior to surgery.

Management of acute maxillary sinusitis post-sinus lift surgery involves a reassessment of the integrity of the soft tissue closure and whether the graft is infected. A 2-week course of antibiotics and debulking of thc graft with proper soft tissue closure is often necessary if there is suppuration and a foul odour from the infection. Occasionally, a buccal fat pad flap has to be mobilised to endure an intact seal of the sinus from the oral cavity. Sinusitis resulting from maxillary sinus augmentation is considered a Class 1 sinonasal complication according to Felisati classification and should be addressed surgically with a combined endoscopic endonasal and endoral approach [33].

4.11.3 Other Complications

Other procedure-related risks include:

- Facial infection.
- Inflammation and pain.
- Injury to the infraorbital nerve resulting in altered sensation of the face.
- Scar formation affecting sinus drainage.
- Bleeding and hematoma formation.
- Graft failure and resorption.
- Oro-antral perforation and fistula.
- Tilting or loosening of implants with extrusion through the wound closure.
- Implant displacement into the sinus (Fig. 4.18).

When such complications arise, the patient must be treated in a timely fashion in order to reduce implant failure and prevent chronic sequelae. The otolaryngologists are the primary specialists that can deal with sinus disease and should be consulted if necessary. This collaboration will increase the likelihood of a better procedural outcome and also provide a good medicolegal cover in event of complications [14].

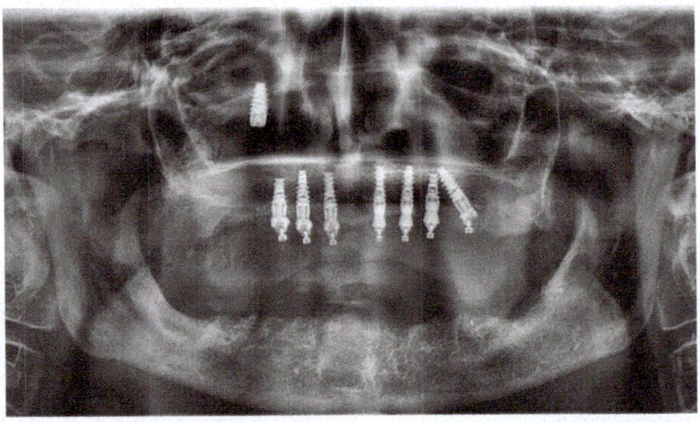

Fig. 4.18 Upper right molar implant displaced into the maxillary sinus. Patient was asymptomatic, and this was discovered only prior to implant exposure for prosthodontic restoration

4.12 Alternative Techniques to Sinus Lift

There are some alternative techniques to sinus augmentation. Horizontal and vertical augmentation using onlay block grafts can be attempted but with less success [14]. Implants can also be placed in a posteriorly angulated direction to avoid the maxillary sinus [34] or bypassing fixation in the alveolar bone and engaging the zygoma [35].

The use of short implants (4–8 mm long) is a simple alternative to sinus augmentation and longer implants. This alternative is potentially less complex, cheaper and faster. There has been research comparing this alternative to sinus augmentation and longer implants. The current short-term evidence does not seem to indicate any difference in implant failure rate between the two groups [30].

References

1. Sharan A, Madjar D. Maxillary sinus pneumatization following extractions: a radiographic study. Int J Oral Maxillofac Implants. 2008;23(1):48–56.
2. Boyne PJ, James RA. Grafting of the maxillary sinus floor with autogenous marrow and bone. J Oral Surg. 1980;38:613–6.
3. Tatum H. Maxillary and sinus implant reconstructions. Dent Clin N Am. 1986;30(2):207–29.
4. Summers RB. A new concept in maxillary implant surgery: the osteotome technique. Compend Contin Educ Dent. 1994;15:152–8.
5. Aimetti M, Massei G, Morra M, Cardesi E, Romano F. Correlation between gingival phenotype and schneiderian membrane thickness. Int J Oral Maxillofac Implants. 2008;23:1128–32.
6. Pommer B, Dvorak G, Jesch P, Palmer RM, Watzek G, Gahleitner A. Effect of maxillary sinus floor augmentation on sinus membrane thickness in computed tomography. J Periodontol. 2012;83(5):551–6.
7. Rosano G, Taschieri S, Gaudy JF, Del Fabbro M. Maxillary sinus vascularization: a cadaveric study. J Craniofac Surg. 2009;20(3):940–3. https://doi.org/10.1097/SCS.0b013e3181a2d77f.
8. Elian N, Wallace S, Cho SC, Jalbout ZN, Froum S. Distribution of the maxillary artery as it relates to sinus floor augmentation. Int J Oral Maxillofac Implants. 2005;20(5):784–7.
9. Heitz-Mayfield LJ, Huynh-Ba G. History of treated periodontitis and smoking as risks for implant therapy. Int J Oral Maxillofac Implants. 2009:24(Suppl):39–68.
10. Pjetursson BE, Tan WC, Zwahlen M, Lang NP. A systematic review of the success of sinus floor elevation and survival of implants inserted in combination with sinus floor elevation. J Clin Periodontol. 2008;35(8 Suppl):216–40. https://doi.org/10.1111/j.1600-051X.2008.01272.x.
11. Esposito M, Grusovin MG, Rees J, Karasoulos D, Felice P, Alissa R, Worthington H, Coulthard P. Effectiveness of sinus lift procedures for dental implant rehabilitation: a cochrane systematic review. Eur J Oral Implantol. 2010;3(1):7–26.
12. Handschel J, Simonowska M, Naujoks C, Depprich RA, Ommerborn MA, Meyer U, Kübler RN. A histomorphometric meta-analysis of sinus elevation with various grafting materials. Head Face Med. 2009;5:12. https://doi.org/10.1186/1746-160X-5-12.
13. Esposito M, Grusovin MG, Felice P, Karatzopoulos G, Worthington HV, Coulthard P. Interventions for replacing missing teeth: horizontal and vertical bone augmentation techniques for dental implant treatment. Cochrane Database Syst Rev. 2009;4:CD003607.
14. Pignataro L, Mantovani M, Torretta S, Felisati G, Sambataro G. ENT assessment in the integrated management of candidate for (maxillary) sinus lift. Acta Otorhinolaryngol Ital. 2008;28(3):110–9.

15. Yang HM, Bae HE, Won SY, Hu KS, Song WC, Paik DJ, Kim HJ. The buccofacial wall of maxillary sinus: an anatomical consideration for sinus augmentation. Clin Implant Dent Relat Res. 2009;11(Suppl 1):e2–6. https://doi.org/10.1111/j.1708-8208.2009.00138.x.
16. Barone A, Santini S, Marconcini S, Giacomelli L, Gherlone E, Covani U. Osteotomy and membrane elevation during the maxillary sinus augmentation procedure. A comparative study: piezoelectric device vs. conventional rotative instruments. Clin Oral Implants Res. 2008;19(5):511–5. https://doi.org/10.1111/j.1600-0501.2007.01498.x.
17. Choi KS, Kan JY, Boyne PJ, Goodacre CJ, Lozada JL, Rungcharassaeng K. The effects of resorbable membrane on human maxillary sinus graft: a pilot study. Int J Oral Maxillofac Implants. 2009;24(1):73–80.
18. García-Denche JT, Wu X, Martinez PP, Eimar H, Ikbal DJ, Hernández G, López-Cabarcos E, Fernandez-Tresguerres I, Tamimi F. Membranes over the lateral window in sinus augmentation procedures: a two-arm and split-mouth randomized clinical trials. J Clin Periodontol. 2013;40(11):1043–51. https://doi.org/10.1111/jcpe.12153.
19. Suárez-López Del Amo F, Ortega-Oller I, Catena A, Monje A, Khoshkam V, Torrecillas-Martínez L, Wang HL, Galindo-Moreno P. Effect of barrier membranes on the outcomes of maxillary sinus floor augmentation: a meta-analysis of histomorphometric outcomes. Int J Oral Maxillofac Implants. 2015;30(3):607–18. https://doi.org/10.11607/jomi.3886.
20. Wen SC, Lin YH, Yang YC, Wang HL. The influence of sinus membrane thickness upon membrane perforation during transcrestal sinus lift procedure. Clin Oral Implants Res. 2015;26(10):1158–64.
21. Jensen SS, Terheyden H. Bone augmentation procedures in localized defects in the alveolar ridge: clinical results with different bone grafts and bone-substitute materials. Int J Oral Maxillofac Implants. 2009;24(Suppl):218–36.
22. Kim Y-K, Cho Y-S, Yun P-Y. Assessment of dentists' subjective satisfaction with a newly developed device for maxillary sinus membrane elevation by the crestal approach. J Periodontal Implant Sci. 2013;43(6):308–14. https://doi.org/10.5051/jpis.2013.43.6.308.
23. Pjetursson BE, Rast C, Brägger U, Schmidlin K, Zwahlen M, Lang NP. Maxillary sinus floor elevation using the (transalveolar) osteotome technique with or without grafting material. Part I: implant survival and patients' perception. Clin Oral Implants Res. 2009;20(7):667–76. https://doi.org/10.1111/j.1600-0501.2009.01704.x.
24. Chen L, Cha J. An 8-year retrospective study: 1,100 patients receiving 1,557 implants using the minimally invasive hydraulic sinus condensing technique. J Periodontol. 2005;76(3):482–91.
25. Troedhan A, Kurrek A, Wainwright M. Biological principles and physiology of bone regeneration under the schneiderian membrane after sinus lift surgery: a radiological study in 14 patients treated with the transcrestal hydrodynamic ultrasonic cavitational sinus lift (intralift). Int J Dent. 2012;2012:576238. https://doi.org/10.1155/2012/576238.
26. Kfir E, Kfir V, Eliav E, Kaluski E. Minimally invasive antral membrane balloon elevation: report of 36 procedures. J Periodontol. 2007;78:2032–5.
27. Kim YK, Lee JY, Park JW, Kim SG, Oh JS. Sinus membrane elevation by the crestal approach using a novel drilling system. Implant Dent. 2017;26(3):351–6. https://doi.org/10.1097/ID.0000000000000570.
28. Palmer P, Palmer R. Implant surgery to overcome anatomical difficulties. In: Palmer R, editor. A clinical guide to implants in dentistry. London: British Dental Association; 2000. p. 57–65.
29. Valentin-Opran A, Wozney J, Csimma C, Lilly L, Riedel GE. Clinical evaluation of recombinant human bone morphogenic protein-2. Clin Orthop Relat Res. 2002;395:110–20.
30. Pinchasov G, Juodzbalys G. Graft-free sinus augmentation procedure: a literature review. J Oral Maxillofac Res. 2014;5(1):e1.
31. Esposito M, Felice P, Worthington HV. Interventions for replacing missing teeth: augmentation procedures of the maxillary sinus. Cochrane Database Syst Rev. 2014;5:CD008397. https://doi.org/10.1002/14651858.CD008397.pub2. Review.
32. Katranji A, Fotek P, Wang HL. Sinus augmentation complications: etiology and treat- ment. Implant Dent. 2008;17:339–49.

33. Felisati G, Chiapasco M, Lozza P, Saibene AM, Pipolo C, Zaniboni M, Biglioli F, Borloni R. Sinonasal complications resulting from dental treatment: outcome oriented proposal of classification and surgical protocol. Am J Rhinol Allergy. 2013;27(4):e101–6. https://doi.org/10.2500/ajra.2013.27.3936.
34. Aparicio C, Perales P, Rangert B. Tilted implants as an alternative to maxillary sinus grafting: a clinical, radiologic, and periotest study. Clin Implant Dent Relat Res. 2001;3:39–49.
35. Esposito M, Worthington HV. Interventions for replacing missing teeth: dental implants in zygomatic bone for the rehabilitation of the severely deficient edentulous maxilla. Cochrane Database Syst Rev. 2013;9:CD004151.
36. Kqiku L, Biblekaj R, Weiglein AH. Location of the extraosseous and intraosseous arterial anastomosis of the maxillary sinus in edentulous specimens. Clin Oral Investig. 2016;20(8):2311–4.

Iliac Crest Graft

5

Thomas Mücke and Stephan Haarmann

5.1 Introduction

Bone grafts are widely used since 1920 for the purpose of oral and maxillofacial surgery. Especially for defect reconstruction during the First and Second World War, its use is well described and was successfully performed in lots of patients. For mandibular reconstruction or augmentation, the first use of this transplant is not well documented, but it is assumed that in the same period as mentioned above, it has been frequently applied for this purpose as well.

Interestingly, there are several donor sites available with different advantages and disadvantages (Table 5.1) [1, 2]. Although the donor sites are quite common and especially established in different centers from a historically point of view, its grafting depends mainly on the type of surgical treatment and the experience of the surgical team [3]. If, for example, a patient needs a complex surgery at the head because of a trauma of the midface and a coronary approach is necessary, a graft from the skull is easily accessible and suitable for reconstruction of the orbital floor if necessary [4]. In contrast, this type of graft may be dangerous considering the risk of injury of the dura if the surgical team is not experienced with this donor site and might damage both outer and inner part of the skull bone during extraction with a bit [4]. One of the main advantages using the iliac crest for bone grafting is its variable form and amount at the anterior and/or posterior part of the iliac crest [5–7]. In addition, both sites are available and can be used non-vascularized or vascularized for further microsurgical reconstructions. If necessary, even both variants can be

T. Mücke (✉)
Department Oral Maxillofacial-Plastic Surgery, Malteser Clinic, St. Josefshospital, Krefeld-Uerdingen, North Rhine-Westphalia, Germany

Department of Oral and Maxillofacial Surgery, Technische Universität München, Klinikum rechts der Isar, Munich, Germany

S. Haarmann
Private Practice of Oral, Maxillofacial and Plastic Surgery, Lippstadt, Germany

A. S. Budihardja, T. Mücke (eds.), *Bone Management in Dental Implantology*,
https://doi.org/10.1007/978-3-319-78951-4_5

Table 5.1 Comparison of different bone grafts with its parts and volumina available for grafting purposes

Donor site	Possible graft forms	Maximal volume available (ml)
Extraoral		
Posterior iliac crest	Block and/or spongiform	140
Anterior iliac crest	Block and/or spongiform	70
Tibia	Spongiform	20–40
Skull	Block	40
Intraoral		
Vertical mandible	Block	5–10
Anterior mandible	Block and/or spongiform	5
Tuber maxillae	Spongiform	2

applied in one patient from one donor site only, microsurgically, and free iliac crest reconstruction at the same time. This should be also implemented in the surgical planning if a possible microsurgical reconstruction is possibly needed in the future in case of unsuccessful treatment by non-vascularized iliac crest grafts.

The grafts of the iliac crest are well documented scientifically and clinically, providing a high amount of bone available for harvesting [6, 7]. With transplantation of such bone, the surgeon is able to shape the harvested bone in the form and position necessary, especially considering the prosthetic position of the abutment [5]. The bone is, because of its individual character, not associated with foreign antigens ande therefore not problematic due to inflammative reactions or host-versus-graft reactions. The grafts include in general vital and non-vital parts, allowing for an induction of the bone as well as conduction of growth, while remodeling processes occur. These characteristics allow for fast and reliable healing if the bone is covered by soft tissue. The biological behavior and the mechanic characteristics are well described. As this graft is taken from the patient, no additional costs have to be considered neither for taking this graft nor for processing after this graft has been taken [8]. It is therefore cheap, but not associated with any disadvantages in case of inflammation as the grafts are simply resorbed and do not need a complete removement, a problem well known with bone xenografts or synthetic bone grafts [8].

Disadvantages with this bone grafts are the necessary donor site morbidity and another wound at the patient's body at a different site than the oral cavity [9]. There are several possibilities for complications at the donor site, especially bleeding which occurs most often and should be critically assessed in the postoperative period. The closing of the wound should be performed very meticulous and exact regarding tissues and layers above the iliac crest. Another disadvantage is the unclear stability of the bone during the healing process [9]. Extensive resorption might be a problem over a time period longer than 6 weeks of healing, making a second grafting and augmentation necessary.

The storage of the bone harvested is possible for the surgical treatment only; further storage is not recommended. Infections as well as cell devitalization should be considered if storage time is prolonged. The medium in which the harvested bone is embedded should be blood kept from the donor site or a medium with electrolyte and energy substrate. Dry storage should be avoided. In addition, the time between harvest and application on the transplanted site should be as short as possible. A major point remains the coverage with soft tissue, which can and should be prepared before bone augmentation.

5.2 Clinical Assessment and Planning

The type of bone, either blocks or spongiform parts, for harvesting should be adopted to the prosthetic and surgical planning [2, 5, 10, 11]. For sinus augmentation in the upper jaw, which seems to be suitable in case of less soft tissue available and extended maxillary sinuses, spongiform parts are favored and recommended [10, 11]. If soft tissue is available and the patient needs reconstruction of the alveolar ridge for different reasons, block techniques in addition with spongiform parts should be considered for stable augmentative results. By using monocortical blocks, the shape of the augmented bone can be individually formed [5]. This aids for a large amount of augmentation and avoids displacement of spongiform parts, which might be reasonable for wound healing disturbances. Blocks should be therefore stabilized by at least two screws, but three are recommended for avoiding displacement. In case of spongiform parts of the iliac crest, fibrin glue can be used for stabilization as well. If this is not available, stable blood components might be processed for further stabilization but do not allow the same stability compared with fibrin glue.

After successful application of transferred bone grafts, a healing period of 6 weeks is recommended until implants might be inserted. After 6 weeks the bone is stable in most cases on the one hand, and on the other hand, bone remodeling processes are still active, allowing for perfect healing of implants after this time period. Another advantage of this short term is that bone resorption of transferred bone has not taken place, yet, but would happen after this time period. General recommendations include a 3-month period of healing of the bone after bone augmentation. The authors experience with a short term is very good, but individual changes of this concept, especially if patients received previous radiotherapy, might be reasonable and safer changing and prolonging the treatment plan of bone healing.

5.3 Surgical Approach

The surgical approach is mostly very easy in case if the patient does not have obesity or previous operations at the donor site. Normally, the posterior part of the iliac crest is preferred due to stability and surgical access reasons. Another advantage is that the scar is not very exposed in the posterior region and postoperative care and avoiding of infections are easier. The iliac crest is examined and palpated. The best option in our opinion is cutting right above the iliac crest and preparing the subcutaneous fatty tissue straightforward to the periosteum of the iliac crest. Doing so allows seeing any cutaneous nerval branches in case of crossing where the cut has been made [12]. Further, the periosteum is incised sharply with a scalpel and subperiosteal preparation of the bone is performed. The medial part of the iliac crest can be completely used for augmentative procedures, either monocortical or in combination with the lateral part as a bicortical graft [6, 7]. Further spongiosa can be gained without any problems. It is meticulous after bone grafting that adequate bleeding control is performed [6]. We recommend the use of bone wax and collagen material for avoidance of bleedings. In addition, it should be a drainage applied into the situs for measurements and control of possible bleedings. We normally use a drain of 10 in size or bigger, which can be removed on the first postoperative day. For illustration of the procedure, see Fig. 5.1.

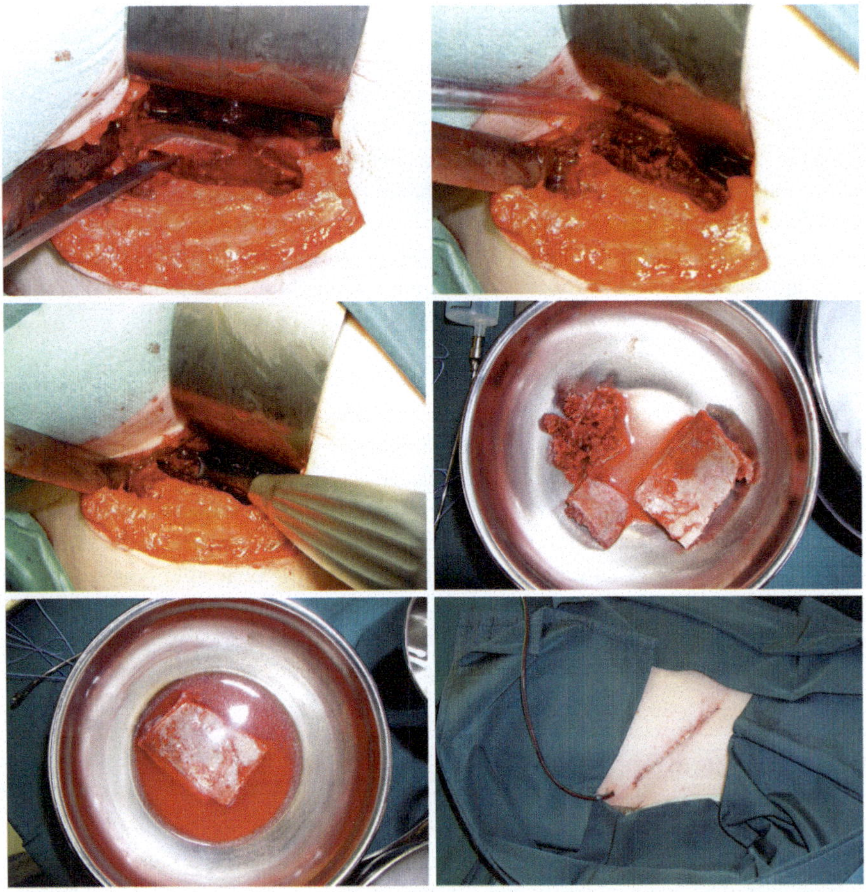

Fig. 5.1 The gaining of monocortical bone graft in combination with spongiosa is illustrated. After the easy access through skin, fat, and fascia is performed, the bone can be easily divided at the medial portion of the posterior iliac crest. This can be performed with a saw or even with a bit, as illustrated here. The spongiform part of the iliac crest is exposed and makes further gaining easily possible. In the right middle picture, you can see the result after gaining, which allows for extensive augmentative procedures. Take care of the bone, and use the blood of the patient with Ringer's solution for storage. At the end, you can see the closure in combination with a drain (size 12)

5.3.1 Cases with Augmentation

Spongioplasty can be used for both internal and external augmentations. It is well known that the effect of preparation of the Schneiderian membrane is the most important step in the preparation of the internal part, reducing the space of the sinus. In this step, it is meticulous that the membrane is left intact. If this is the case, spongiosa is a well-known and established material for internal augmentation. In addition, a lateral augmentation can make sense for further reconstruction of the atrophied alveolar ridge. The following case makes this procedure more clear (Figs. 5.2, 5.3, 5.4, 5.5, and 5.6).

The internal augmentation can also performed alone or in addition with the external augmentation using cortical bone in combination with spongiosa for contouring. In this context it is important that bone margins should be avoided supporting the healing process. Especially soft tissue healing can be affected by sharp bone and should be therefore protected during healing.

The application or treatment with implants should be performed after 6–12 weeks after augmentation, as the bone is still in process of healing. It is mandatory that no wound healing disturbances occurred. The following case illustrates the complete procedure of augmentation and implantation with a follow-up of 6 years postoperatively.

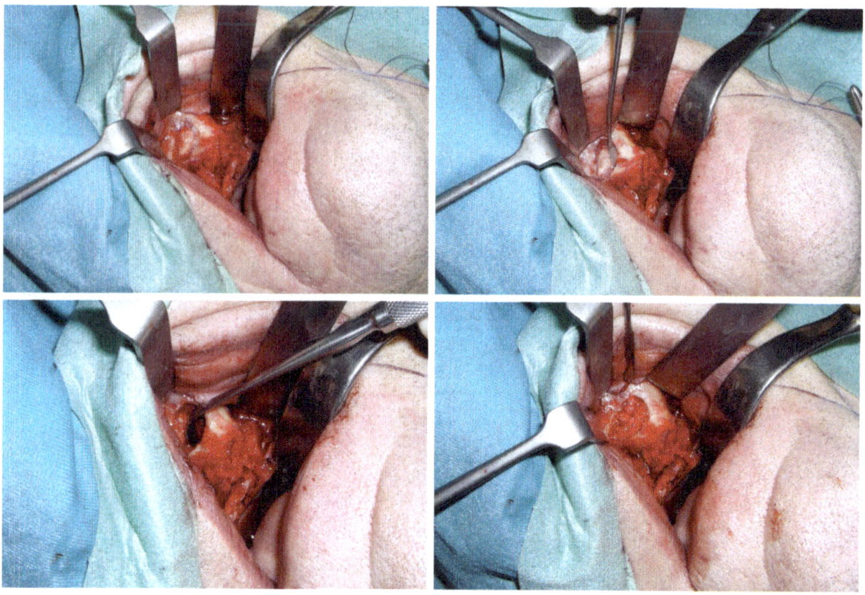

Fig. 5.2 After exposure of the maxilla, the membrane of the sinus is exposed and carefully prepared from the bone. After elevation of the membrane without any damage, spongiosa is used for internal augmentation

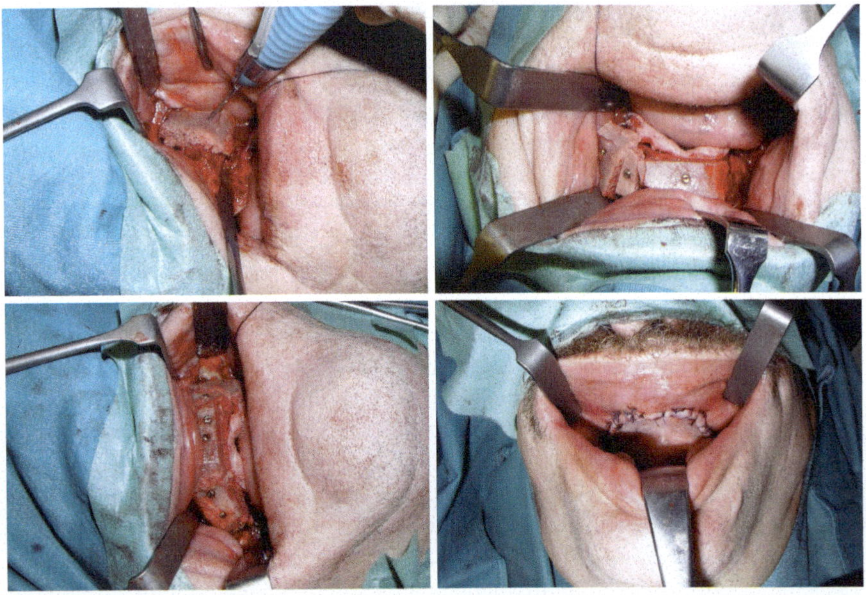

Fig. 5.3 Same patient as illustrated before with additional lateral augmentation. After the first monocortical blocks have been fixed by at least two screws, spongiosa is used for further contouring. The margins of the blocks were smoothed and accurate wound closure was performed

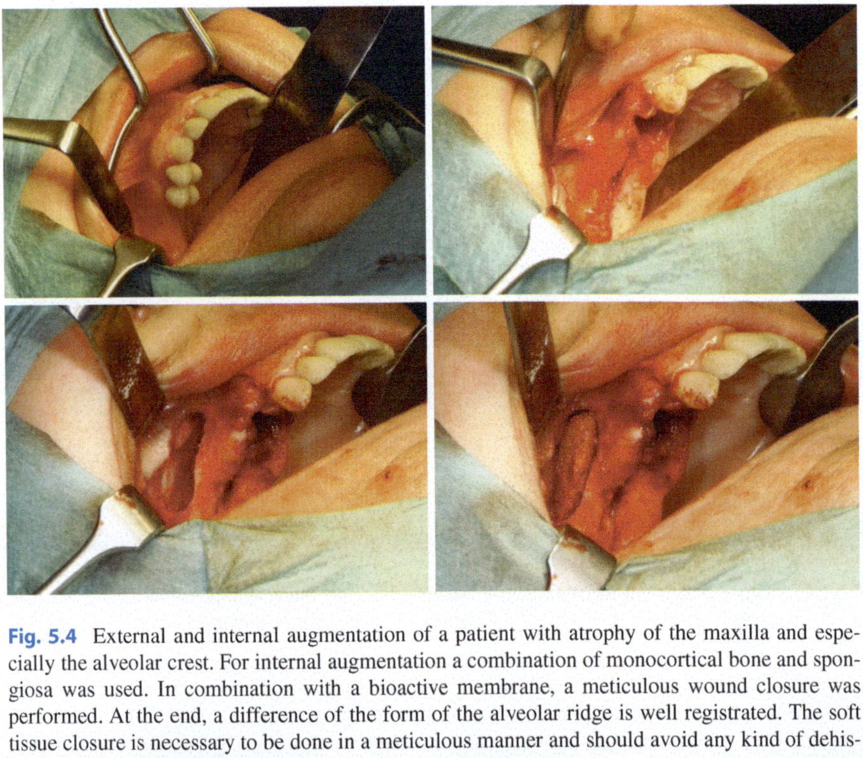

Fig. 5.4 External and internal augmentation of a patient with atrophy of the maxilla and especially the alveolar crest. For internal augmentation a combination of monocortical bone and spongiosa was used. In combination with a bioactive membrane, a meticulous wound closure was performed. At the end, a difference of the form of the alveolar ridge is well registrated. The soft tissue closure is necessary to be done in a meticulous manner and should avoid any kind of dehiscence in the postoperative course

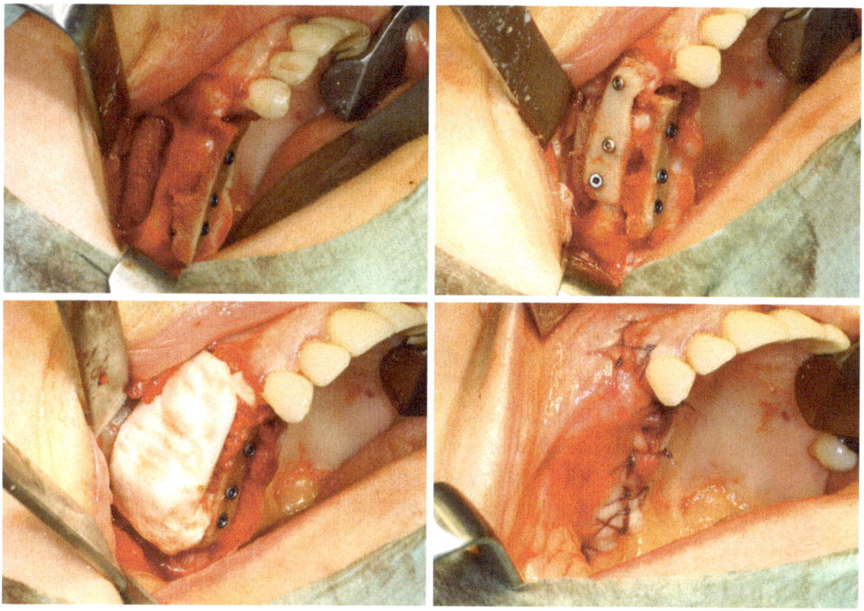

Fig. 5.4 (continued)

5.3.2 Complications

After bone transplantation, either by spongioplasty or block augmentations, the most probable complications are exposure of the augmented bone and wound healing disturbances at the recipient site or even infections [9, 13]. All these complications can be easily avoided or managed by a 5-day postoperative course with intravenous antibiotic treatment [13]. The first few days, especially between days 1 and 3 postoperatively, are the most vulnerable time for these complications [9, 13, 14]. In this time span, it remains absolutely necessary that the bone is not exposed and the patients should be informed that eating and speaking are dangerous for mechanical reasons. A nasogastric tube is often recommended avoiding mechanical stress by the food during eating by the patient [9]. We considered using fibrin glue in addition to the regular spongioplasties for stabilization of the bone and fixation underneath the mucosal layer. It may be discussed that using fibrin glue might be a barrier for the postoperative healing, but we did not have any major complication by using the glue. In case that the mucosa is dehisence, the glue might be helpful in the secondary wound healing and the fixation of the spongiform bone mass.

Minor complications at the iliac crest remain hematoma formation or seromas [13–15]. Although these complications are not clinically relevant for the healing itself, patients are often impaired severely due to the regular postoperative follow-ups, which are necessary for supporting the healing and control of possible infections [9, 14]. Active bleedings can occur in the postoperative course within 2 days and might be severe and underestimated, since the iliac crest includes a large space

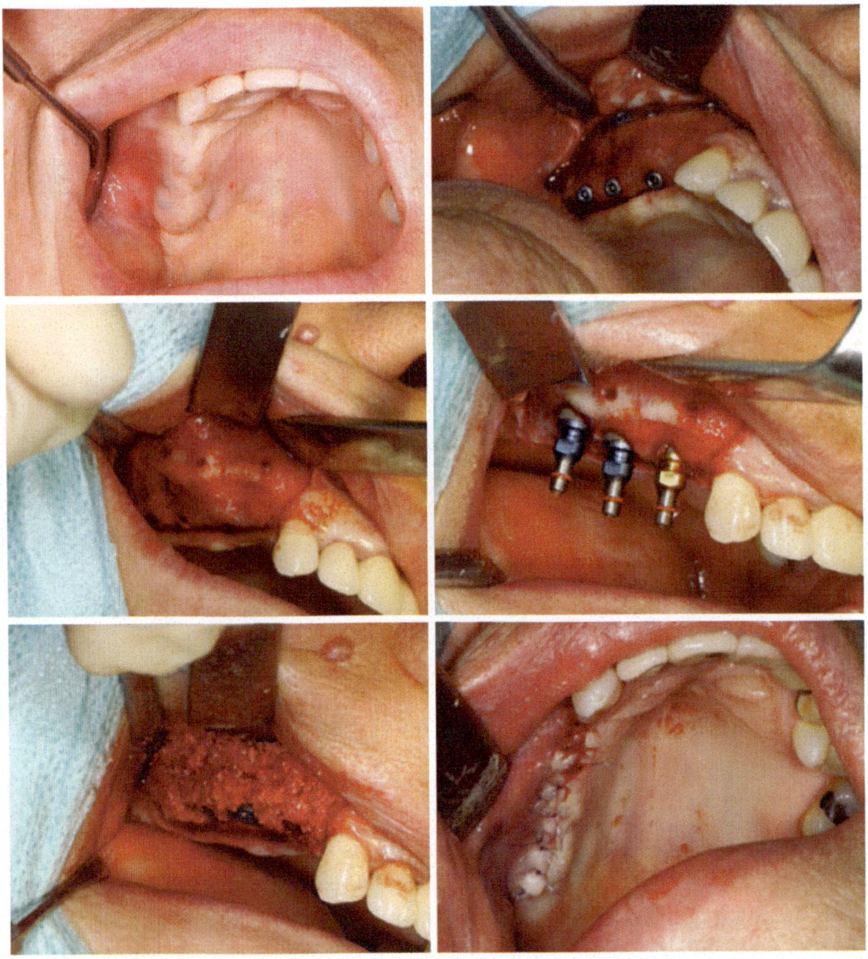

Fig. 5.5 Same patient as before after 12 weeks of wound and bone healing. The first picture illustrates the uneventful healing process with the intact mucosa. The next picture shows the healed augmented bone suitable for implantation. After removal of the fixing screws, implants were inserted in a preplanned position, considering the prosthetic treatment afterward. The bone gained after the implants was inserted according to the manufacture's protocol was used for additional lateral augmentation

to the medial site, which can be overlooked or hardly examined by the unexperienced colleague. This complication is a very dangerous and important major complication which can be life-threatening in severe cases as well. Therefore, ultrasound or dedicated clinical observation in the postoperative period for 2 days is mandatory [14, 15].

Rare complications include fractures of the iliac crest (Fig. 5.7) or in case of incorrect bone grafting fractures involving more than the iliac crest including the

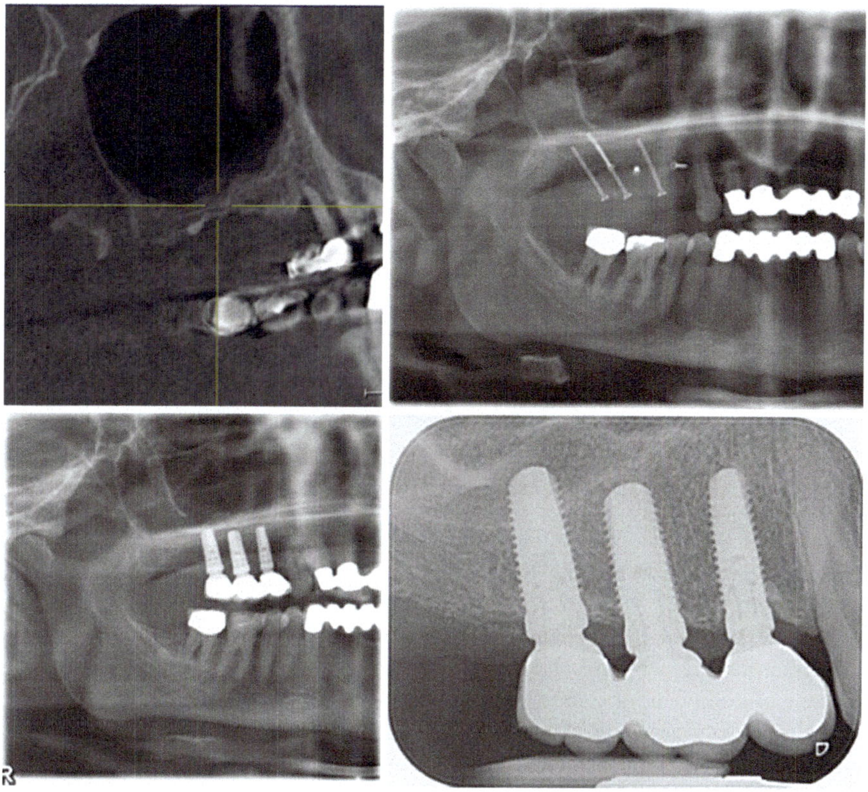

Fig. 5.6 Radiographs showing the treatment course over a treatment follow-up postoperatively after implant insertion of 6 years. The initial situation showed the minimal bone height, making internal and external augmentations necessary for a sufficient bone level suitable for implantation. After anchorage of the iliac crest grafts, a well-formed alveolar crest became visible with the fixing screws, illustrated by the panoramic overview. The result after implant insertion and prosthetic treatment shows a well-planned dental rehabilitation. The last picture illustrates the result of implantation as well as the prosthetic treatment after 6 years. The bone cannot be differed between iliac crest graft or orthotopic maxillary bone structure

pelvic. In some cases the superior spine of the iliacal part can be fractured although the operative site can be not associated with this part (Fig. 5.7). In these cases a refixation should be considered. In addition, herniation can also occur in case of unsuccessful wound closure at the donor site [16]. This can be easily avoided by correct closure of the layers and dedicated suturing of muscle structures and periosteal parts [16].

In general, more complications might occur at this donor site as well as at the recipient site, but these are most often not important for the patient or surgeon. It is important that the patient is observed and examined in the postoperative period [13–15].

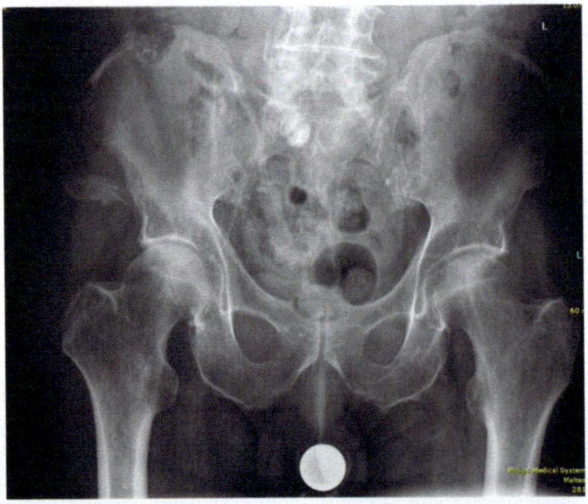

Fig. 5.7 Complication after bone grafting at the right iliac crest. Although the donor site for bone grafting is not associated with the superior spine, a fracture occurred at day 8 postoperatively with involvement of the complete spine. The patient had a defect reconstruction with non-vascularized bicortical iliac crest and suffered from osteoporosis

5.3.3 Special Considerations

The authors would like to emphasize that iliac bone grafts are well described, important for augmentative and reconstructive surgery in the maxillofacial region. In case of complications, these grafts are resorbed in parts or completely if the infection is severe or prolonged. In contrast to synthetic bone materials, the iliac crest is included into the bone available at the recipient site and allows for long-term survival and stabilization. Synthetic or allogenic grafts have to be removed mostly in case of infections. It should be also considered that the bone graft should be taken in a non-vascularized way from a site allowing for microvascular bone grafting from the other site. This includes that the ipsilateral iliac crest at a defect at the lower lateral mandible is preserved. We chose mostly spongiform grafts but also monocortical and bicortical blocks for reconstruction of the alveolar ridge, especially considering its form and further prosthetic treatments.

References

1. Castagna L, Polido WD, Soares LG, Tinoco EM. Tomographic evaluation of iliac crest bone grafting and the use of immediate temporary implants to the atrophic maxilla. Int J Oral Maxillofac Surg. 2013;42:1067–72.
2. Dhawan A, Kuklo TR, Polly DW Jr. Analysis of iliac crest bone grafting process measures. Am J Orthop (Belle Mead NJ). 2006;35:322–6.
3. Kolomvos N, Iatrou I, Theologie-Lygidakis N, Tzerbos F, Schoinohoriti O. Iliac crest morbidity following maxillofacial bone grafting in children: a clinical and radiographic prospective study. J Craniomaxillofac Surg. 2010;38:293–302.
4. Scheerlinck LM, Muradin MS, van der Bilt A, Meijer GJ, Koole R, Van Cann EM. Donor site complications in bone grafting: comparison of iliac crest, calvarial, and mandibular ramus bone. Int J Oral Maxillofac Implants. 2013;28:222–7.

5. Kademani D, Keller E. Iliac crest grafting for mandibular reconstruction. Atlas Oral Maxillofac Surg Clin North Am. 2006;14:161–70.
6. Kilinc A, Korkmaz IH, Kaymaz I, Kilinc Z, Dayi E, Kantarci A. Comprehensive analysis of the volume of bone for grafting that can be harvested from iliac crest donor sites. Br J Oral Maxillofac Surg. 2017;55:803–8.
7. Zhu SS, Feng G, Li JH, Luo E, Hu J. Correction of mandibular deficiency by inverted-L osteotomy of ramus and iliac crest bone grafting. Int J Oral Sci. 2012;4:214–7.
8. Pirris SM, Nottmeier EW, Kimes S, O'Brien M, Rahmathulla G. A retrospective study of iliac crest bone grafting techniques with allograft reconstruction: do patients even know which iliac crest was harvested? Clinical article. J Neurosurg Spine. 2014;21:595–600.
9. Fretwurst T, Wanner L, Nahles S, Raguse JD, Stricker A, Metzger MC, et al. A prospective study of factors influencing morbidity after iliac crest harvesting for oral onlay grafting. J Craniomaxillofac Surg. 2015;43:705–9.
10. Cobb AR, McCarthy E, Van Zyl M, Ayliffe PR. Alveolar bone grafting: use of the Jacob's chuck with trephine to harvest iliac crest cancellous bone. Br J Oral Maxillofac Surg. 2011;49:239–40.
11. Constantinides J, Chhabra P, Turner PJ, Richard B. A comparison of Shepard's osteotome versus trapdoor flap technique to harvest iliac crest bone for secondary alveolar bone grafting. Cleft Palate Craniofac J. 2008;45:347–52.
12. den Brave PS, Vas Nunes SE, Bronkhorst MW. Anatomical variations of the lateral femoral cutaneous nerve and iatrogenic injury after autologous bone grafting from the iliac crest. J Orthop Trauma. 2015;29:549–53.
13. Matsa S, Murugan S, Kannadasan K. Evaluation of morbidity associated with iliac crest harvest for alveolar cleft bone grafting. J Maxillofac Oral Surg. 2012;11:91–5.
14. Loeffler BJ, Kellam JF, Sims SH, Bosse MJ. Prospective observational study of donor-site morbidity following anterior iliac crest bone-grafting in orthopaedic trauma reconstruction patients. J Bone Joint Surg Am. 2012;94:1649–54.
15. Lementowski PW, Lucas P, Taddonio RF. Acute and chronic complications of intracortical iliac crest bone grafting versus the traditional corticocancellous technique for spinal fusion surgery. Orthopedics. 2010;33:PMID:20415304.
16. Ou CJ, Sternfeld WC, Stausmire JM. Iliac crest herniation secondary to autogenous bone grafting found on osteopathic examination. J Am Osteopath Assoc. 2015;115:518–21.

Vascularized Bone Grafts

6

Thomas Mücke

6.1 Introduction

Reconstructive surgery in the treatment of the head and neck region has been improved over the recent decades by the routine use of free flap reconstruction and refining microvascular techniques [1]. The reconstruction of bony defects due to trauma, deformities, or tumor-associated defects including cysts and either benign or malignant defects after resection in the head and neck area presents a challenge to the surgeon for both functional and aesthetic reasons. The basic principle of reconstruction is to rebuild anatomical structures with bone and soft tissue as similar as possible to that found in the area of origin. To reach these aims, the surgeon requires optimal tissues to reconstruct the defect area. These defects can be reconstructed either by local or microvascular flaps. Local flaps and especially non-vascularized bone grafts are suitable for reconstruction of small defects which will not and did not yet receive radiation. Local flaps but also microvascular flaps can be combined with avascular bone grafts in case that the bone graft is not bigger than 3–5 cm in length with a well-vascularized wound bed in which the bone, most frequently iliac crest grafts, can be embedded. Although this technique is often successful, with the development of reliable microvascular free flap reconstruction, several flaps are available for a good functional and aesthetic outcome with the option to withstand irradiation [2].

These free composite flaps can provide a sufficient bone length and reliable wound healing even at complicated recipient sites. The scapula [3], iliac crest [4], and fibula [5–7] are all well-established donor sites with an adequate amount of tissues and good-quality corticocancellous bone which can be contoured by

T. Mücke (✉)
Department Oral Maxillofacial-Plastic Surgery, Malteser Clinic, St. Josefshospital, Krefeld-Uerdingen, North Rhine-Westphalia, Germany

Department of Oral and Maxillofacial Surgery, Technische Universität München, Klinikum rechts der Isar, Munich, Germany

A. S. Budihardja, T. Mücke (eds.), *Bone Management in Dental Implantology*,
https://doi.org/10.1007/978-3-319-78951-4_6

osteotomies and allows anchorage of dental implants allowing for complete reconstruction and rehabilitation [8]. In recent years the fibula osteocutaneous flap has become increasingly a standard method for reconstruction in the mandible [9]. Several authors favor this flap over the scapula and iliac crest flap [10] for reconstruction: the patients have less donor-site morbidity [11], and the length offers a better possibility for excellent contouring. The perforators of the peroneal artery permit the inclusion of a reliable skin paddle in the fibula flap for better soft tissue reconstruction [10]. Especially development of 3D techniques for planning the shape and cutting of the fibula flap as well as the planned resection or reconstruction of defects enhanced the procedure with a benefit for both the surgeon and patients [12–17]. This tool allows for a faster surgical procedure with a high accuracy and predictable result [14, 16], even possible with intraoperative implantation in a previously planned position [18]. On the other hand, the iliac bone crest flap offers a high amount of bone available for complex reconstructions in the dentate mandible [19]. The microvascular iliac crest can also be planned virtually previously [20–22] including all advantages and disadvantages of virtual planning [23–28]. Both these flaps can be harvested using the widely recognized "two-team" approach, thus minimizing operating time, expense, and patient morbidity. They are thus the most widely used composite free flaps in head and neck reconstruction, as the scapula flap or the osteocutaneous radial forearm flap is associated with more disadvantages in comparison with these two microvascular flaps containing a large amount of bone with little morbidity.

A comparison between the microvascular iliac crest and fibular free flap revealed the different overall complication and success rates in a prospective study [29]. The relations between wound infection, microvascular revisions, and free flap failure in patients requiring bony microsurgical reconstruction were significantly different distributed in two similar cohorts [29]. In addition, the occurrence and type of postoperative complications was significantly associated with the type of bony free flap used for reconstruction, with a worse outcome for iliac crest flaps [29]. This shows that the fibular free flaps with an additional skin paddle are generally favored because of the possible shaping and adopting to the form of the mandible or maxilla for reconstruction [30]. Although both flaps are suitable for reconstruction of the jaws and allow for dental rehabilitation, the wound closure is always meticulous for further healing and overall success rate of bony reconstruction [29–31].

The overall success rate of free flaps in the literature, either soft tissue or bony flaps, is within the range of iliac crest and fibula flaps [1, 29, 32], although the overall success rates of all free flaps are generally higher than in osseous free flaps only. The success rate of free flaps overall is very high between 94% and 97% [1, 32, 33], even in patients with a prior history of oncologic or reconstructive treatments [1, 33]. Although these studies have included soft and osseous free flaps, they demonstrate the high validity of microvascular reconstructions. In contrast, bony reconstructions of the jaws are generally associated with a higher complication rate, especially in situations with wound infections at the recipient site [32–34], in case of osteomyelitis due to irradiation or antiresorptive agents [35]. The negative influence of wound infections and revisions on overall flap success has been described before [33, 34]. The role of infection is of particular interest in patients after complex surgical operations [1]. In addition, in patients with previous radiotherapy, infections are common and associated with free flap failure [33] putting the whole procedure at risk [1, 33, 36].

For bony reconstruction and dental rehabilitation by implant insertion within the microvascular free flap, the fibula flap and the iliac crest flap are both well suited for a complete reconstruction, including all steps until the patient is able to eat and chew. Both types of free flaps are associated with advantages and disadvantages, which are often obvious but sometimes dangerous for the result, if the planning is not considered in detail. Especially the site of harvesting is of crucial importance for the reconstructive result, as well as the presence of suitable vessels for microvascular anastomosis [29, 33].

The shaping of the fibula is one of the advantages described in the literature, but also prolonged overall operation time is described as a possible disadvantage [37]. The flexibility of the skin paddle is another advantage of the fibular free flap but also is time-consuming due to the handling of the skin paddles containing small perforators [38–40]. Nevertheless, the fibula flap is associated with significantly fewer complications such as infections at the recipient site and free flap loss compared to the iliac crest flap [29]. Cordeiro reported no free flap losses in a retrospective study over 10 years evaluating 135 free fibular and three iliac crest flaps [41]. Due to this data, the fibular flap was favored by this group [41]. In contrast, Rogers et al. found a higher complication rate at the donor site of this flap in these patients compared with the iliac crest flap reconstruction, evaluated by functional and quality-of-life evaluation after free flap reconstructions of the mandible [42]. Interestingly, anastomosis of both microvascular arterial flap vessels of the fibular or iliac crest flap to the facial artery was a significant risk factor for flap failure [29]. For this reason, alternative recipient vessels may be chosen for microvascular anastomosis. In this chapter, we would like to emphasize both advantages and disadvantages of the fibular free flap as well as the iliac crest flap. In addition, alternative concepts are also presented to understand the concept of microvascular free flaps in the field of bony reconstructions.

6.2 Clinical Assessment and Planning

6.2.1 Microvascular Fibula Free Flap

This flap should be always controlled before harvesting by using angiography of the legs, investigating the anatomy of the patient, and considering possible complications in the nutrition of the legs. If there are venous insufficiency of arterial plaques with disruption of the arteries, another flap should be considered.

The fibula flap can be harvested easily due to the reliable vessel diameter and the correct method of harvesting. Although the harvesting procedure is prolonged, because perforator vessels should be identified and preserved, there are some important advantages and disadvantages as follows.

6.2.1.1 Advantages

The main advantage of this kind of flap remains the variable design, which can be achieved by using this flap. The length and quality of bone is very outstanding and allows for maxillary and mandible reconstruction, as well as a very comfortable bone for implantation purposes. The bone is suitable for all kind of wound beds, especially if soft tissue is necessary after bony reconstruction. This skin is directly placed over the bone for reconstruction, which is also a very important argument in case of a difficult reconstruction. The length and shape of the fibula flap allows for 2–4 segments which can be used for reconstruction of the mandible, especially if extended defects are present. The donor-site morbidity is quite low in case of an accurate and successful defect coverage of the skin, if this is needed for further coverage of the bone.

6.2.1.2 Disadvantages

The most important disadvantage of this flap remains the obvious scar and frequently occurring wound healing disturbances. Although for skin replacement full-thickness skin grafts or split-thickness skin grafts are conventionally used, these grafts often show displacements or unsuccessful healing. Secondary wound management is then often necessary. Another disadvantage of this flap is the required experience, especially in flap planning for reconstruction but also for raising of this flap. In some patients discomfort at the ankle function-wise is reported. This has to be considered in the choice of this flap.

6.2.2 Microvascular Iliac Crest Flap

This flap constantly allows for a large amount of bone and includes reliable vessels which are constantly present at its origin in the iliac region. There is no need for preoperative evaluations of vessels, but the microvascular anastomoses are somewhat more challenging compared with the fibula flap.

The iliac crest flap can be harvested easily due to the exposed region in thin patients and the correct method of harvesting. Traditionally, this flap is frequently used in the UK, as this flap is one of the standard free flaps taught in the training program and provides well-perfused bone. Although the harvesting might be faster compared with the fibula flap, the pedicle of the flap is more sensible that the pedicle of the fibula flap and monitoring is more difficult. We normally use this kind of flap without using a skin island, which has been frequently described as reliable, but in clinical practice, the skin is often compromised and should be well considered. In cases with the need for additional soft tissues, a fibula free flap is favored, since this skin paddle is variable in size form and shaping is also easier, because it is more robust in handling. In summary, there are some important advantages and disadvantages of the iliac crest flap as follows.

6.2.2.1 Advantages

The main advantage of this flap remains the high amount of bone available for reconstruction, allowing for a safe dental rehabilitation and facial reconstruction if the perfusion is well achieved. Another advantage is the possible two-team approach and the direct primary closure of the donor site without the need for additional skin from another site. The resulting scar is also not affecting the patient aesthetic-wise or functional-wise. Ipsilateral use of the iliac crest contains also a very similar form and shape of the mandibular angle region to the paramandibular region or of the maxilla of the same site. Therefore, implant placement is simplified by the shape, form, and amount of bone if correctly osteosynthesized and positioned according to the corresponding jaw.

6.2.2.2 Disadvantages

The most important disadvantage of this flap remains the lower success rated due to the sensible pedicle of the flap which cannot be monitored by simple or cheap methods. Vessel spasm is more frequently present compared with other flaps with comparative possibilities. One very difficult disadvantage and possible confounder remains the higher frequency of bleedings from the muscle cuff of the flap or the bone itself, resulting in possible pedicle pressure and compromise of flap perfusion. At this time we would like to emphasize that the use of bone wax and consequent coagulation of muscle bleedings should be performed to avoid these complications. Another typical but less frequent disadvantage which has been described is hernia formation at the abdominal wall and can be easily avoided by dedicated wound closure. In some cases sensory loss might be present at the lateral femoral region but is well tolerated by the patient.

6.3 Surgical Approach

6.3.1 Microvascular Fibula Flap

The fibular free flap can be harvested as described [31, 43–45]; we prefer always including a skin paddle, which is helpful for monitoring but also for soft tissue management in the coverage of the flap. The landmarks, the head of the fibula and the lateral malleolus, are of importance. Behind the posterior border of the fibula, the perforator vessels nourishing the skin paddle course in the posterior septum (Fig. 6.1).

The skin incision should be performed on the fibula bone itself or a little bit more anterior, depending on the amount and size of additional tissue and skin needed for reconstruction. After the skin is incised and the underlying fat and fascia is also cut, the muscle becomes visible. The skin is completely incised over the whole length as planned and the septum inspected. The perforators located in the posterior septum should be carefully prepared. These perforator vessels are also possible to be used as pure perforator flaps (Fig. 6.2).

After preparation of the fibula straight on the bone, the peroneus muscle should be removed from the bone and the posterior margin containing the septum strictly

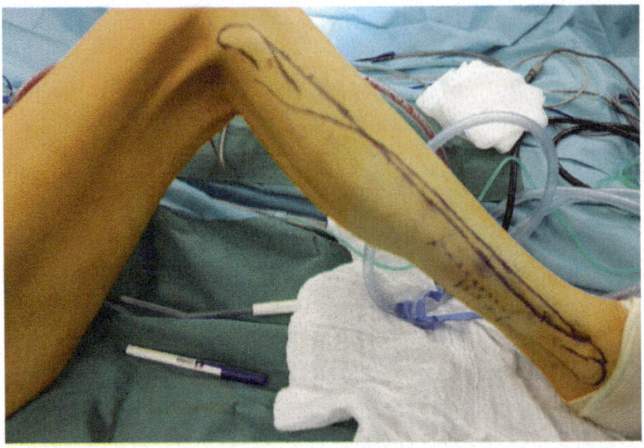

Fig. 6.1 Landmarks of the fibula flap are marked and the skin paddle with possible perforator vessels identified by Doppler or ICG angiography

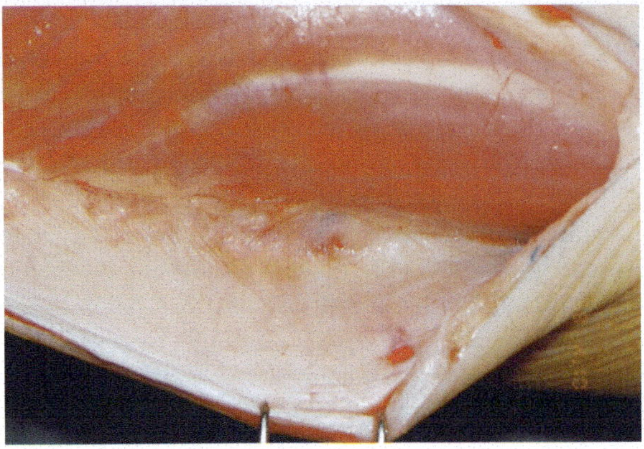

Fig. 6.2 Perforator vessels identified at the distal third of the fibula, at the posterior septum, prepared as a perforator flap for reconstruction

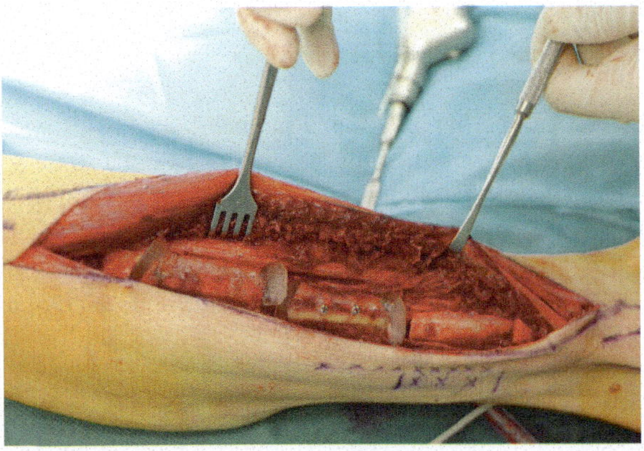

Fig. 6.3 Figure illustrating the fibula segments used for a total mandible reconstruction. The cutting guides are used for immediate reconstruction of the neomandible at the leg after preparation of the bone including a perforator for soft tissue reconstruction. The fibula is used for complete reconstruction of three segments, replacing the mandible from both angles of the mandible

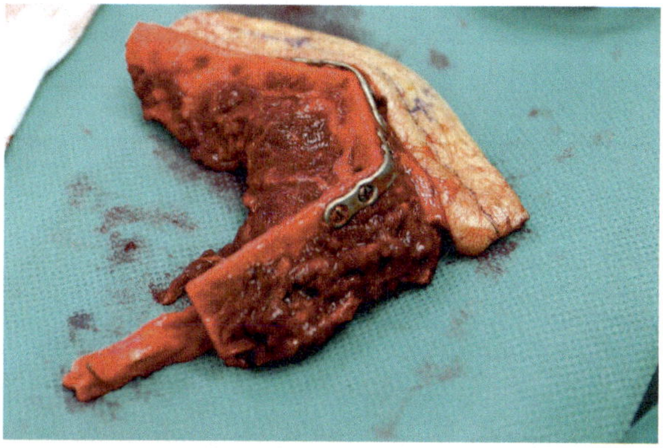

Fig. 6.4 Direct reconstruction of the mandible using cutting guides at the leg and immediate reconstruction while raising the flap for complete mandible reconstruction. The skin with the perforator is planned for soft tissue reconstruction. After completion of osteosynthesis at the leg, the neomandible fits due to the planning perfectly with the help of preplanned cutting guides

preserved. We use to apply cutting guides on the bone for guided and planned reconstruction, especially if mandible or maxillary reconstructions include more than one segment of bone (Fig. 6.3).

After the segments have been cut and the vessels have been prepared for the microvascular anastomosis by identifying the pedicle of the flap, the bone is osteotomized and shaped with the help of the cutting guides. These guides are created by previously virtually planned mandible analysis and 3D planning of the exact positions of osteotomies of the mandible. Doing so is extremely helpful in the intraoperative setting as the time used previously can be saved at the time of the operation. Exact planning is helpful for the flap raising as well, because the osteosynthesis can be performed at the leg while the flap is raised and a second team is still preparing the vessels at the neck. By this two-team approach, the time of anesthesia is reduced for the patient, and the resection or reconstruction of the maxilla or mandible can be exactly reproduced with the help of the cutting guides. The flap can be shaped and fits normally exactly in the preplanned position (Fig. 6.4).

The fibula flap allows for a two-team approach, raising the flap simultaneously to the preparation of the defect region including the preparation of potential microvascular vessels for anastomosis at the neck. The shape of the fibula flap is very helpful for reconstructions, especially if the patients want to receive dental implants in the follow-up time. If the fibula flap contains to less bone, it can be easily augmented by additional use of iliac crest spongioplasty. The bone is very helpful if the patient needs some more bone in cases with a good mouth opening,

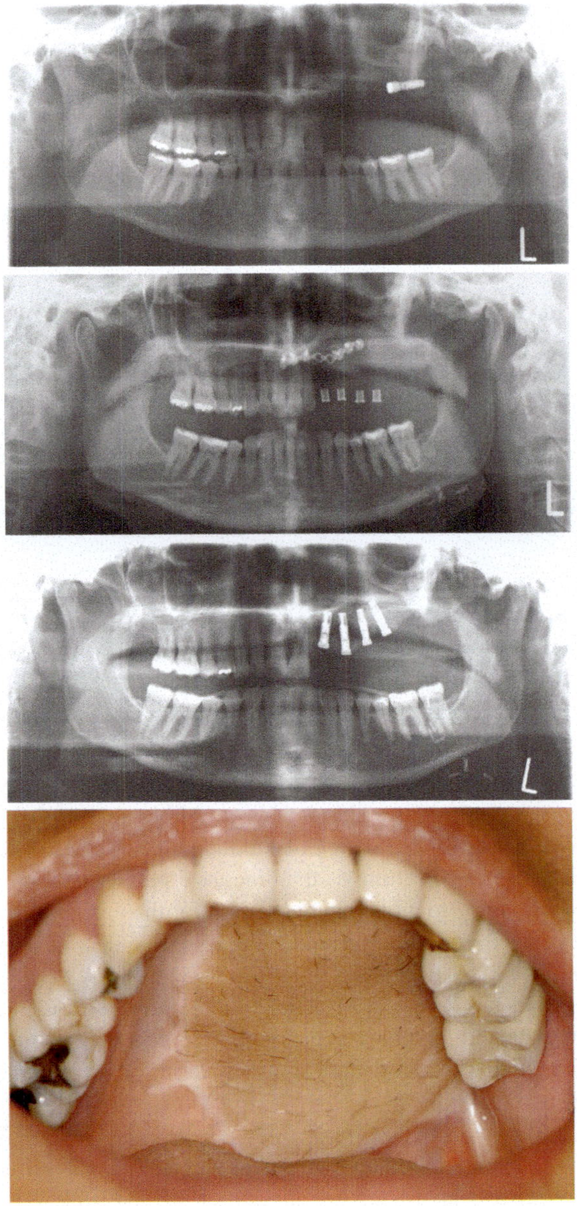

Fig. 6.5 Case illustration showing a complete dental rehabilitation using a microvascular fibula flap in the maxilla. Starting from a zygoma implant without any function or even possible loading, the patient was reconstructed by an osteocutaneous fibula flap including closure of the oroantral fistula. Then, implants were planned after thinning the skin island and loaded by a functional dental prosthesis

but careful acting should be included into considerations if previous radiation therapies have been applied. Then, less bone might be more helpful because the mouth opening is reduced and prosthetic treatments are often very difficult in such situations (Fig. 6.5).

6.3.2 Microvascular Iliac Crest Flap

The iliac crest flap has been already well described in the literature [45, 46]. The region of the flap should be investigated before planning, and previous operations at this site should be carefully considered. We always excluded sites where spongioplasties have been performed but already include this consideration at the first indication for spongioplasty if possible. Although small mandible or maxillary defects due to different reasons might be no problem at first sight, it should be avoided using the ipsilateral site for harvesting spongiosa as the "easy" defect can also be caused by a malignant disease like central squamous cell carcinomas, ameloblastomas, or other entities. Therefore, we always exclude the ipsilateral site for spongioplasties, having still the choice of microvascular iliac crest transfer in the following.

Surgically, the anterior spina iliaca superior and the pubic tubercle should be identified, following the course of the inguinal ligament (Fig. 6.6). As the supplying artery, the superficial circumflex iliac artery, arises from the femoral artery, we plan

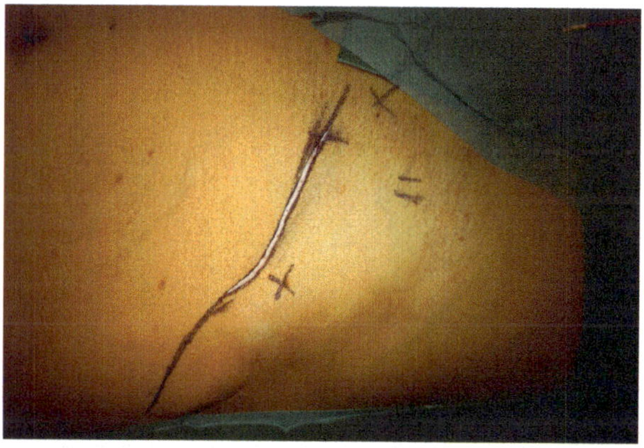

Fig. 6.6 The incision is performed after identifying the landmarks of the flap. The inguinal ligament is considered and its course also included into the planning of the incision

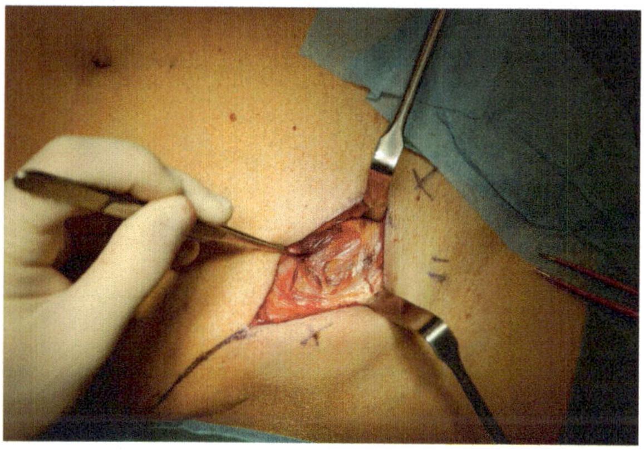

Fig. 6.7 After incision of the skin and identifying the inguinal ligament, the preparation is continued in direction to the femoral artery and vein. The muscle is divided and the vessels can be subsequently prepared after exposure of the layers underneath the external oblique muscle fibers

to identify the femoral artery first and second the arising superficial circumflex artery. A major advantage using this way is that the femoral artery can be easily palpated and the superficial circumflex iliac artery is reliably identified without any accidental damage. The artery can be achieved by 2 cm incision above the inguinal ligament and subsequent exposure of the subcutaneous tissue, following to the femoral artery. The external oblique muscle can be exposed underneath the subcutaneous fat tissue and incised according to the fibers' course (Fig. 6.7).

At the time of identifying the muscle, possible perforators nourishing the skin can be also identified, but normally we avoid including a skin paddle. By subsequent exposure of the internal oblique muscle fibers (and also the transversalis muscle in parts), a fascia will become visible and should be incised to exposure the superficial circumflex iliac artery (Fig. 6.8).

The course of the vessels is followed carefully to the lateral aspect of the situs achieving the iliac region. At this site, the muscle parts at the superior anterior iliac

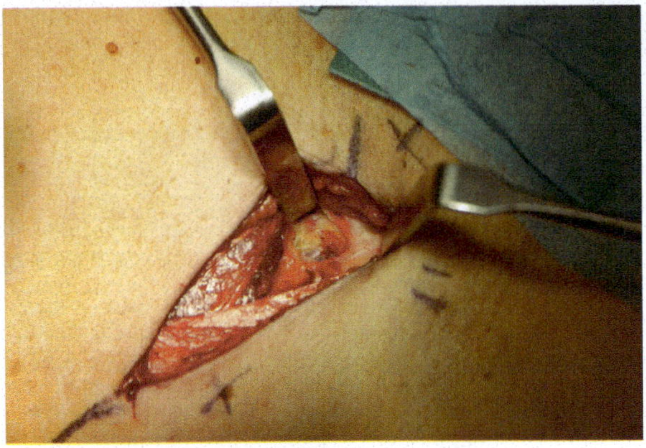

Fig. 6.8 Identification of the vascular pedicle (superficial circumflex iliac artery and deep circumflex iliac vein) of the iliac crest flap after incision of the internal muscle fibers and the fascia underneath these fibers. The pedicle is exposed close to the femoral artery and vein

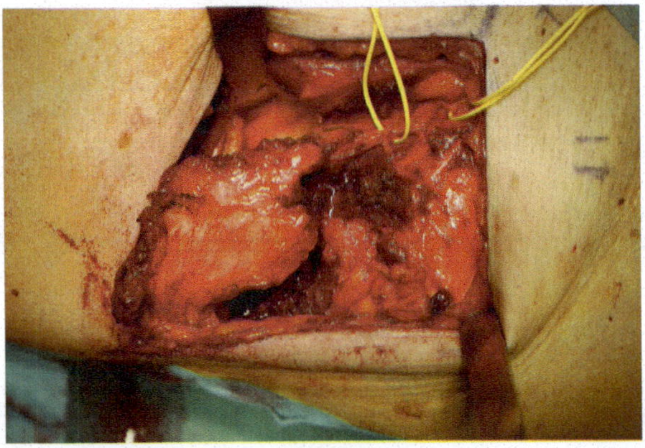

Fig. 6.9 Identification of the vascular pedicle (including superficial circumflex iliac artery and deep circumflex iliac vein) and following its course after the surrounding muscles from the iliac crest is mandatory and should be prepared. After this has been done the bone is exposed. At this time it is generally recommended to reduce the amount of muscle as the flap becomes too bulky if the muscle cuff is not consequently reduced

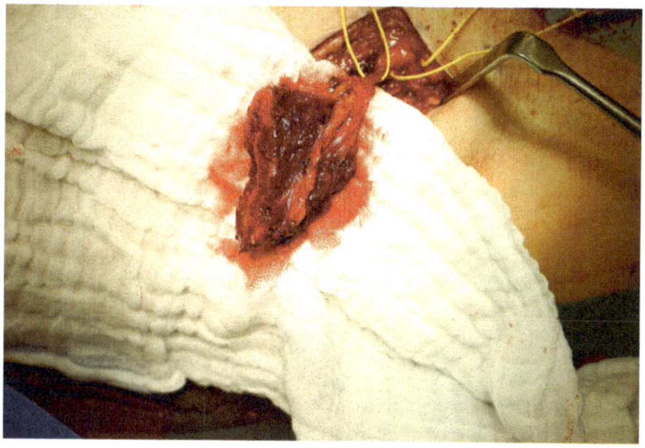

Fig. 6.10 Completion of flap raising after the osteotomy is completed including the suitable amount of bone. Note the bleedings from muscle and bone

spine are left intact, and the iliac crest should be further exposed. At the lateral part of the iliac crest, the muscles can be completely separated without any problems. The pedicle is not at risk at this site. The iliac crest at the medial site should be carefully exposed after identification of the pedicle (Fig. 6.9).

At this stage, the osteotomy of the bone should be performed to complete the raising of the flap. The pedicle of this flap is normally short and a ligation should be put safely at the vessels' origin (Fig. 6.10).

6.4 Complications

Most complications have already been described at the time of explaining possible disadvantages. The most important and complicated event is free flap loss resulting in a defect, which should be considered for another microvascular reconstruction, or, alternatively, by reconstruction of a local or pedicled flap (e.g., pectoralis major flap). The occurrence of complications is quite high and includes also functional impairments like sensory or motoric loss of function. The frequency of wound healing disturbances at the fibula site is quite high, and general medical complications (e.g., lung infection) also occur frequently. Rogers et al. found a higher complication rate at the donor site of the fibula flap in these patients compared with the iliac crest flap reconstruction, evaluated by functional and quality-of-life evaluation after free flap reconstructions of the mandible [42]. Interestingly, anastomosis of both microvascular arterial flap vessels of the fibular or iliac crest flap to the facial artery was a significant risk factor for flap failure [29]. The facial vein was also shown to be an independent risk factor for the fibular flap for flap loss [29]. A higher risk for microsurgical revision was also detected if the artery of the flap was anastomosed to the facial artery. Although the anastomosis to the facial artery is generally supposed to be very safe [47], contradictory data is also reported in the literature [29]. Operation time, if very long, was a risk factor for free flap loss in this study; however this is entirely intuitive and probably unavoidable as it acts as an indicator of the complexity of the case as well as the difficulty of surgery [29].

6.5 Special Considerations

Bony reconstruction allows the use of osseointegrated implants for functional dentition when adequate bone stock is replaced [19, 48, 49]. In comparison to other bone grafts, the fibula osteocutaneous flap and the iliac crest flap seem to be the best options in facial reconstruction for different reasons [50]. Both flaps provide bone dimensions consistently adequate for implant placement [8, 51]. Because of its size and form, the deep circumflex iliac artery flap has for many years been the most popular method for reconstruction of facial bone defects [4, 52, 53]. Extensive soft tissue coverage can be achieved with skin and muscle from the iliac region. The height of the harvested bone enables the surgeon to insert implants easily and reliably with a high rate of success [4, 8, 53, 54]. However, postoperative pain and complications have made the flap unpopular among surgeons in some regions of the world.

The fibula osteocutaneous flap can lead to satisfactory results both functionally and aesthetically over a long period of time [3, 10, 48, 50, 55–60]. This flap is not only an ideal approach for the reconstruction of mandibular defects [5, 11, 44, 50, 51, 59, 61–64]; it is also an excellent graft for the reconstruction of maxillary defects. The advantages of the flap are the sufficient bone length, the long pedicle, the amount of harvestable skin up to 14 × 25 cm [11, 60, 62, 63], and the low donor-site morbidity [5, 8, 11, 48, 58, 60, 63, 65, 66]. Moreover, in comparison with the bulky iliac crest, soft tissue management can be accomplished easily. Thinning of the applied tissue is precisely possible with a pleasant result which is, because of the bulky surrounding, superior to the management of the iliac crest. The bicortical bone provides reliable stability and a low rate of bone atrophy [44, 54, 67]. The height of the fibula can be increased by using the double-barrel technique which is already a standard method for increasing the supply of bone [44, 68].

In our opinion reconstruction with one free vascularized bone graft and further insertion of osteointegrated implants with teeth is the most advantageous solution for patients with defects of the jaws. Even small bone defects are appropriate for this kind of treatment because the risk of resorption, infection, and osteomyelitis can aggravate the primary situation. When complications occur, multiple surgical procedures prolong the time needed for recovery. The length, quality, and nearly constant amount of bone in long-term follow-up in combination with its long pedicle and versatile skin paddle make it ideal for reconstruction in several cases. The goal of total oral rehabilitation and restoration, both functionally and aesthetically, can be achieved only by using the fibula osteocutaneous or iliac crest flap in a reliable way to prevent asymmetric contours of the middle and lower face. Owing to the suitable bone graft of the fibula flap, implants can be inserted and improve the functional and aesthetic appearance of the midface by employing single-tooth restoration or with implant-supported prostheses if necessary. Nevertheless, the requirements of the wound need to be carefully matched to the characteristics of the appropriated flap prior to the reconstructive procedure.

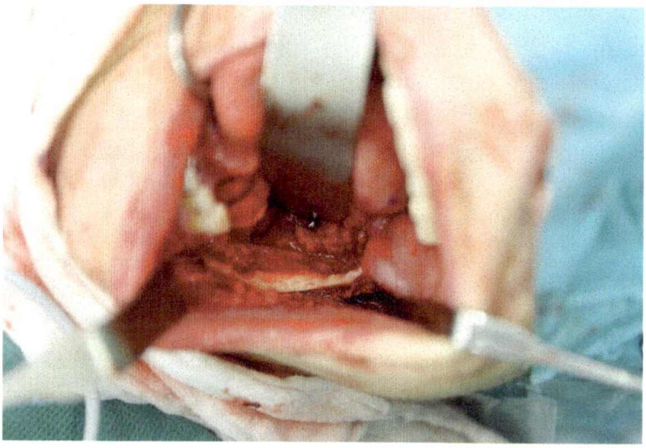

Fig. 6.11 Defect containing bone and soft tissue after a complex tumor surgery with the aim of full dental rehabilitation in an 85-year-old woman. A rim resection has been performed

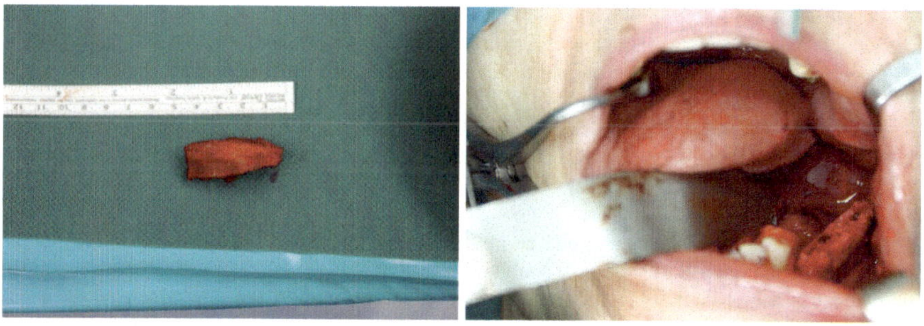

Fig. 6.12 After harvesting of the bone block, an osteosynthesis was performed using two screws for alveolar ridge reconstruction

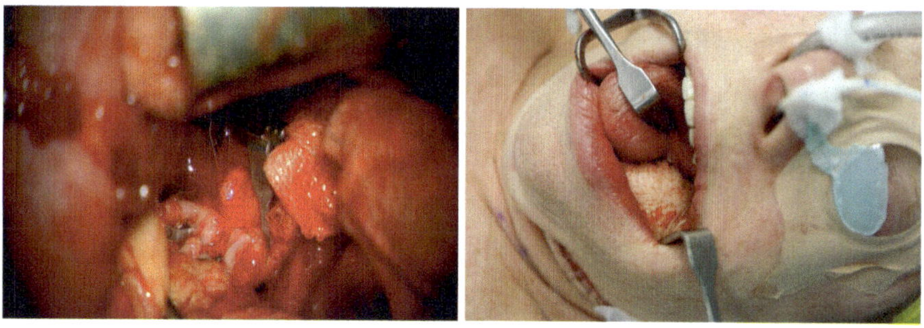

Fig. 6.13 After completion of intraoral microvascular anastomosis of the perforator flap to the facial artery and vein (left figure), the flap was inserted into the oral cavity and the bone covered (right figure)

A combination of techniques as reported in this book is also a reliable and suitable option. The possibility of avascular bone blocks in combination with a microvascular free flap can be performed in some cases if appropriate. The combination can be considered in patients at higher ages or if contraindications for a microvascular free flap like the fibula flap (e.g., not three vessels present at the leg) are present. Previous operations at the possible donor site are also one reason for changing to his type of concept. The following case illustrates the use of a microvascular anterolateral perforator flap with intraoral anastomosis in combination with a free iliac crest block graft (Fig. 6.11, 6.12, and 6.13).

This case shows the variability and possibilities of methods applicable for bone reconstructions even in extensive or difficult situations.

References

1. Mücke T, Wolff KD, Wagenpfeil S, Mitchell DA, Hölzle F. Immediate microsurgical reconstruction after tumor ablation predicts survival among patients with head and neck carcinoma. Ann Surg Oncol. 2010;17:287–95.
2. Liu YM, Chen GF, Yan JL, Zhao SF, Zhang WM, Zhao S, et al. Functional reconstruction of maxilla with pedicled buccal fat pad flap, prefabricated titanium mesh and autologous bone grafts. Int J Oral Maxillofac Surg. 2006;35:1108–13.
3. Swartz WM, Banis JC, Newton ED, Ramasastry SS, Jones NF, Acland R. The osteocutaneous scapular flap for mandibular and maxillary reconstruction. Plast Reconstr Surg. 1986;77:530–45.
4. Riediger D. Restoration of masticatory function by microsurgically revascularized iliac crest bone grafts using enosseous implants. Plast Reconstr Surg. 1988;81:861–77.
5. Hidalgo DA. Fibula free flap: a new method of mandible reconstruction. Plast Reconstr Surg. 1989;84:71–9.
6. Taylor GI, Miller GD, Ham FJ. The free vascularized bone graft. A clinical extension of microvascular techniques. Plast Reconstr Surg. 1975;55:533–44.
7. Wales CJ, Morrison J, Drummond R, Devine JC, McMahon J. Pre-operative evaluation of vascularised fibula donor sites: a UK maxillofacial e-survey. Br J Oral Maxillofac Surg. 2010;48:192–4.
8. Frodel JL Jr, Funk GF, Capper DT, Fridrich KL, Blumer JR, Haller JR, et al. Osseointegrated implants: a comparative study of bone thickness in four vascularized bone flaps. Plast Reconstr Surg. 1993;92:449–55.. discussion 56–8.
9. Foster RD, Anthony JP, Singer MI, Kaplan MJ, Pogrel MA, Mathes SJ. Reconstruction of complex midfacial defects. Plast Reconstr Surg. 1997;99:1555–65.
10. Ferri J, Caprioli F, Peuvrel G, Langlois JM. Use of the fibula free flap in maxillary reconstruction: a report of 3 cases. J Oral Maxillofac Surg. 2002;60:567–74.
11. Kildal M, Wei FC, Chang YM. Free vascularized bone grafts for reconstruction of traumatic bony defects of mandible and maxilla. World J Surg. 2001;25:1067–74.
12. Rana M, Chin SJ, Muecke T, Kesting M, Groebe A, Riecke B, et al. Increasing the accuracy of mandibular reconstruction with free fibula flaps using functionalized selective laser-melted patient-specific implants: a retrospective multicenter analysis. J Craniomaxillofac Surg. 2017;45:1212–9.
13. Eckardt A, Swennen GR. Virtual planning of composite mandibular reconstruction with free fibula bone graft. J Craniofac Surg. 2005;16:1137–40.
14. Rommel N, Kesting MR, Rohleder NH, Bauer FMJ, Wolff KD, Weitz J. Mandible reconstruction with free fibula flaps: outcome of a cost-effective individual planning concept compared with virtual surgical planning. J Craniomaxillofac Surg. 2017;45:1246–50.

15. Roser SM, Ramachandra S, Blair H, Grist W, Carlson GW, Christensen AM, et al. The accuracy of virtual surgical planning in free fibula mandibular reconstruction: comparison of planned and final results. J Oral Maxillofac Surg. 2010;68:2824–32.
16. Schepers RH, Kraeima J, Vissink A, Lahoda LU, Roodenburg JL, Reintsema H, et al. Accuracy of secondary maxillofacial reconstruction with prefabricated fibula grafts using 3D planning and guided reconstruction. J Craniomaxillofac Surg. 2016;44:392–9.
17. Valentini V, Agrillo A, Battisti A, Gennaro P, Calabrese L, Iannetti G. Surgical planning in reconstruction of mandibular defect with fibula free flap: 15 patients. J Craniofac Surg. 2005;16:601–7.
18. Freudlsperger C, Bodem JP, Engel E, Hoffmann J. Mandibular reconstruction with a prefabricated free vascularized fibula and implant-supported prosthesis based on fully three-dimensional virtual planning. J Craniofac Surg. 2014;25:980–2.
19. Brown JS. Deep circumflex iliac artery free flap with internal oblique muscle as a new method of immediate reconstruction of maxillectomy defect. Head Neck. 1996;18:412–21.
20. Zheng L, Lv X, Zhang J, Liu S, Zhang J, Zhang Y. Translating computer-aided design and surgical planning into successful mandibular reconstruction using a vascularized iliac-crest flap. J Oral Maxillofac Surg. 2017;76(4):886–93.
21. Yu Y, Zhang WB, Wang Y, Liu XJ, Guo CB, Peng X. A revised approach for mandibular reconstruction with the vascularized iliac crest flap using virtual surgical planning and surgical navigation. J Oral Maxillofac Surg. 2016;74:1285.1e–e11.
22. Shen Y, Sun J, Li J, Ji T, Li MM. A revised approach for mandibular reconstruction with the vascularized iliac crest flap by virtual surgical planning. Plast Reconstr Surg. 2012;129:565e–6e.
23. Ayoub N, Ghassemi A, Rana M, Gerressen M, Riediger D, Holzle F, et al. Evaluation of computer-assisted mandibular reconstruction with vascularized iliac crest bone graft compared to conventional surgery: a randomized prospective clinical trial. Trials. 2014;15:114.
24. Kniha K, Mohlhenrich SC, Foldenauer AC, Peters F, Ayoub N, Goloborodko E, et al. Evaluation of bone resorption in fibula and deep circumflex iliac artery flaps following dental implantation: a three-year follow-up study. J Craniomaxillofac Surg. 2017;45:474–8.
25. Modabber A, Ayoub N, Bock A, Mohlhenrich SC, Lethaus B, Ghassemi A, et al. Medial approach for minimally-invasive harvesting of a deep circumflex iliac artery flap for reconstruction of the jaw using virtual surgical planning and CAD/CAM technology. Br J Oral Maxillofac Surg. 2017;55:946–51.
26. Modabber A, Gerressen M, Stiller MB, Noroozi N, Fuglein A, Holzle F, et al. Computer-assisted mandibular reconstruction with vascularized iliac crest bone graft. Aesthet Plast Surg. 2012;36:653–9.
27. Modabber A, Mohlhenrich SC, Ayoub N, Hajji M, Raith S, Dds SR, et al. Computer-aided mandibular reconstruction with vascularized iliac crest bone flap and simultaneous implant surgery. J Oral Implantol. 2015;41:e189–94.
28. Mohlhenrich SC, Kniha K, Elvers D, Ayoub N, Goloborodko E, Holzle F, et al. Intraosseous stability of dental implants in free revascularized fibula and iliac crest bone flaps. J Craniomaxillofac Surg. 2016;44:1935–9.
29. Mücke T, Loeffelbein DJ, Kolk A, Wagenpfeil S, Kanatas A, Wolff KD, et al. Comparison of outcome of microvascular bony head and neck reconstructions using the fibular free flap and the iliac crest flap. Br J Oral Maxillofac Surg. 2013;51:514–9.
30. Mücke T, Loeffelbein DJ, Hohlweg-Majert B, Kesting MR, Wolff KD, Hölzle F. Reconstruction of the maxilla and midface—surgical management, outcome, and prognostic factors. Oral Oncol. 2009;45:1073–8.
31. Mücke T, Hölzle F, Loeffelbein DJ, Ljubic A, Kesting M, Wolff KD, et al. Maxillary reconstruction using microvascular free flaps. Oral Surg Oral Med Oral Pathol Oral Radiol Endod. 2011;111:51–7.
32. Wolff KD, Hölzle F, Wysluch A, Mücke T, Kesting M. Incidence and time of intraoperative vascular complications in head and neck microsurgery. Microsurgery. 2008;28:143–6.
33. Mücke T, Rau A, Weitz J, Ljubic A, Rohleder N, Wolff KD, et al. Influence of irradiation and oncologic surgery on head and neck microsurgical reconstructions. Oral Oncol. 2012;48:367–71.

34. Santamaria E, Wei FC, Chen HC. Fibula osteoseptocutaneous flap for reconstruction of osteoradionecrosis of the mandible. Plast Reconstr Surg. 1998;101:921–9.
35. Mücke T, Jung M, Koerdt S, Mitchell DA, Loeffelbein D, Kesting MR. Free flap reconstruction for patients with bisphosphonate related osteonecrosis of the jaws after mandibulectomy. J Craniomaxillofac Surg. 2016;44:142–7.
36. Bourget A, Chang JT, Wu DB, Chang CJ, Wei FC. Free flap reconstruction in the head and neck region following radiotherapy: a cohort study identifying negative outcome predictors. Plast Reconstr Surg. 2011;127:1901–8.
37. Shen Y, Sun J, Li J, Shi J, Ow A. Long-term results of partial double-barrel vascularized fibula graft in symphysis for extensive mandibular reconstruction. J Oral Maxillofac Surg. 2012;70:983–91.
38. Al Qattan MM, Boyd JB. "Mini paddle" for monitoring the fibular free flap in mandibular reconstruction. Microsurgery. 1994;15:153–4.
39. Alkaabi M, Regan PJ, Kelly J, Mc Cann PJ, Ismael TS. Double paddle free fibular flap for reconstruction of the composite facial tumour in patient with Fanconi's anaemia. J Plast Reconstr Aesthet Surg. 2009;62:e471–3.
40. Loeffelbein DJ, Holzle F, Wolff KD. Double-skin paddle perforator flap from the lateral lower leg for reconstruction of through-and-through cheek defect – a report of two cases. Int J Oral Maxillofac Surg. 2006;35:1016–20.
41. Cordeiro PG, Disa JJ, Hidalgo DA, Hu QY. Reconstruction of the mandible with osseous free flaps: a 10-year experience with 150 consecutive patients. Plast Reconstr Surg. 1999;104:1314–20.
42. Rogers SN, Lakshmiah SR, Narayan B, Lowe D, Brownson P, Brown JS, et al. A comparison of the long-term morbidity following deep circumflex iliac and fibula free flaps for reconstruction following head and neck cancer. Plast Reconstr Surg. 2003;112:1517–25.. discussion 26–7.
43. Hölzle F, Ristow O, Rau A, Mücke T, Loeffelbein DJ, Mitchell DA, et al. Evaluation of the vessels of the lower leg before microsurgical fibular transfer. Part I: anatomical variations in the arteries of the lower leg. Br J Oral Maxillofac Surg. 2011;49:270–4.
44. Hölzle F, Watola A, Kesting MR, Nolte D, Wolff KD. Atrophy of free fibular grafts after mandibular reconstruction. Plast Reconstr Surg. 2007;119:151–6.
45. Wolff KD, Hölzle F. Raising of microvascular flaps: a systematic approach. 2nd ed. Berlin: Springer; 2011.
46. Taylor GI, Townsend P, Corlett R. Superiority of the deep circumflex iliac vessels as the supply for free groin flaps. Plast Reconstr Surg. 1979;64:595–604.
47. Hölzle F, Hohlweg-Majert B, Kesting MR, Mücke T, Loeffelbein DJ, Wolff KD, et al. Reverse flow facial artery as recipient vessel for perforator flaps. Microsurgery. 2009;29:437–42.
48. Futran ND, Wadsworth JT, Villaret D, Farwell DG. Midface reconstruction with the fibula free flap. Arch Otolaryngol Head Neck Surg. 2002;128:161–6.
49. Funk GF, Arcuri MR, Frodel JL Jr. Functional dental rehabilitation of massive palatomaxillary defects: cases requiring free tissue transfer and osseointegrated implants. Head Neck. 1998;20:38–51.
50. Hidalgo DA. Aesthetic improvements in free-flap mandible reconstruction. Plast Reconstr Surg. 1991;88:574–85.. discussion 86–7.
51. Zlotolow IM, Huryn JM, Piro JD, Lenchewski E, Hidalgo DA. Osseointegrated implants and functional prosthetic rehabilitation in microvascular fibula free flap reconstructed mandibles. Am J Surg. 1992;164:677–81.
52. Shenaq SM. Reconstruction of complex cranial and craniofacial defects utilizing iliac crest-internal oblique microsurgical free flap. Microsurgery. 1988;9:154–8.
53. Taylor GI. Reconstruction of the mandible with free composite iliac bone grafts. Ann Plast Surg. 1982;9:361–76.
54. Berggren A, Weiland AJ, Dorfman H. The effect of prolonged ischemia time on osteocyte and osteoblast survival in composite bone grafts revascularized by microvascular anastomoses. Plast Reconstr Surg. 1982;69:290–8.

55. Anthony JP, Foster RD, Sharma AB, Kearns GJ, Hoffman WY, Pogrel MA. Reconstruction of a complex midfacial defect with the folded fibular free flap and osseointegrated implants. Ann Plast Surg. 1996;37:204–10.
56. Chang YM, Coskunfirat OK, Wei FC, Tsai CY, Lin HN. Maxillary reconstruction with a fibula osteoseptocutaneous free flap and simultaneous insertion of osseointegrated dental implants. Plast Reconstr Surg. 2004;113:1140–5.
57. Kazaoka Y, Shinohara A, Yokou K, Hasegawa T. Functional reconstruction after a total maxillectomy using a fibula osteocutaneous flap with osseointegrated implants. Plast Reconstr Surg. 1999;103:1244–6.
58. Nakayama B, Matsuura H, Ishihara O, Hasegawa H, Mataga I, Torii S. Functional reconstruction of a bilateral maxillectomy defect using a fibula osteocutaneous flap with osseointegrated implants. Plast Reconstr Surg. 1995;96:1201–4.
59. Peng X, Mao C, Yu GY, Guo CB, Huang MX, Zhang Y. Maxillary reconstruction with the free fibula flap. Plast Reconstr Surg. 2005;115:1562–9.
60. Yim KK, Wei FC. Fibula osteoseptocutaneous free flap in maxillary reconstruction. Microsurgery. 1994;15:353–7.
61. Flemming AF, Brough MD, Evans ND, Grant HR, Harris M, James DR, et al. Mandibular reconstruction using vascularised fibula. Br J Plast Surg. 1990;43:403–9.
62. Jones NF, Monstrey S, Gambier BA. Reliability of the fibular osteocutaneous flap for mandibular reconstruction: anatomical and surgical confirmation. Plast Reconstr Surg. 1996;97:707–16.. discussion 17–8.
63. Wei FC, Chen HC, Chuang CC, Noordhoff MS. Fibular osteoseptocutaneous flap: anatomic study and clinical application. Plast Reconstr Surg. 1986;78:191–200.
64. Wei FC, Seah CS, Tsai YC, Liu SJ, Tsai MS. Fibula osteoseptocutaneous flap for reconstruction of composite mandibular defects. Plast Reconstr Surg. 1994;93:294–304.. discussion 5–6.
65. Futran ND. Retrospective case series of primary and secondary microvascular free tissue transfer reconstruction of midfacial defects. J Prosthet Dent. 2001;86:369–76.
66. Triana RJ Jr, Uglesic V, Virag M, Varga SG, Knezevic P, Milenovic A, et al. Microvascular free flap reconstructive options in patients with partial and total maxillectomy defects. Arch Facial Plast Surg. 2000;2:91–101.
67. Disa JJ, Hidalgo DA, Cordeiro PG, Winters RM, Thaler H. Evaluation of bone height in osseous free flap mandible reconstruction: an indirect measure of bone mass. Plast Reconstr Surg. 1999;103:1371–7.
68. Jones NF, Swartz WM, Mears DC, Jupiter JB, Grossman A. The "double barrel" free vascularized fibular bone graft. Plast Reconstr Surg. 1988;81:378–85.

Bone Substituting Materials in Dental Implantology

7

Ika Dewi Ana

7.1 Terminology and Functions

The need for bone grafting procedure in dental implantology has become more prevalent to enhance the opportunity to salvage major bone loss. In dentistry, bone graft substitution is directed to regenerate bone faster and better to support dental implant. In some cases, bone graft substitution is used to reduce bone atrophy and improve aesthetics, for example, in patient with gum and periodontal diseases, oral and maxillofacial trauma, or loss of a tooth. The frequency of dental implant surgery and the number of fixtures annually placed in Korea, for example, can be estimated based on the data from implant companies, which is around 500,000–800,000 [1]. Many bone graft options are available, including cortical and cancellous autografts and allografts, each of which has specific biological and mechanical properties [2]. Grafts may be described as cortical, cancellous, cortico-cancellous, or osteochondral which is categorized based on the tissue architecture. Autografts (autogenous) can be transferred directly from the donor to recipient site, while allografts are usually modified or preserved to reduce immunogenicity prior to transplantation. The modification processes include freezing, freeze-drying, irradiation, or chemo-modification [3]. Table 7.1 shows bone graft types based on the origin of the grafts [3].

Biological activities of a bone graft are a result of two functions: osteogenesis and mechanical considerations [4]. Osteogenesis possesses synthesized new bone by graft cells or cells of the host [2]. Surface cells which survive with transplantation of either cortical or cancellous grafts can produce new bone [5–7], which in turn is important for the development of callus during early graft incorporation. Because of its large surface area, the cancellous bone has greater potential to form new bone than the cortical bone. Table 7.2 shows properties of bone grafts [4].

I. D. Ana (✉)
Dental Biomedical Sciences Department, Faculty of Dentistry, Universitas Gadjah Mada, Yogyakarta, Indonesia
e-mail: ikadewiana@ugm.ac.id

A. S. Budihardja, T. Mücke (eds.), *Bone Management in Dental Implantology*, https://doi.org/10.1007/978-3-319-78951-4_7

Table 7.1 Bone graft terminology

Type of graft	Tissue transfer	Remarks
Autograft	From one site to another in the same individual	
Allograft	From two genetically different individuals of the same species	
Xenograft	From one species to a member of different species	
Isograft	From one monozygotic twin to the other	Usually done in laboratory experiments with transfer from inbred genetically identical strains of animal

Table 7.2 Comparative properties of bone grafts

Type of graft	Mechanical properties[a]	Osteoconduction	Inductiveness	Osteogenesis graft derived
Autograft				
Cancellous	±	+++	+++	+++
Cortical	+++	++	++	+
Allograft				
Cancellous				
Frozen	±	++	+	–
Freeze-dried	–	++	+	–
Cortical				
Frozen	+++	+	±	–
Freeze-dried	+	+	±	–
Demineralized				
Allogenic	–	+	++	–
Cancellous chips	–	+	++	–

– no activity; ± little activity, + mild activity, ++ moderate activity; +++ significant activity
[a]Mechanical properties are also defined as the graft's ability to confer structural strength

Osteoinduction is bone graft capacity to provide osteogenic potential by stimulating the host to synthesize a new bone. Mesenchymal stem cells recruited to the site will first differentiate into cartilage then into bone-forming cells. Physiologically differentiation into bone-forming cells occurs through the recruitment of graft-derived proteins, which actively drive the process [6]. Osteoconduction is provided by all grafts and biomaterials such as ceramics. The osteoconduction process supplies three-dimensional framework for the ingrowth into the graft of host capillaries, perivascular tissue, and osteoprogenitor cells from the recipient. Incorporation of the graft into host requires the interaction of osteoinduction and osteoconduction, often described as creeping substitution. The process ultimately leads to the replacement of the graft by host bone in a predictable pattern under the influence of load bearing [8]. Bone graft incorporation is a well-balanced mechanism between the graft and the host and includes all the functions of osteogenesis, osteoinduction, and osteoconduction.

The biological process of the bone regeneration involves inflammatory phase resulted into the migration of inflammatory cells and fibroblast into the graft. Formation of hematoma enhances the release of both cytokines and growth factors.

Osteoinduction drives chemotaxis, mitosis, and differentiation of the host osteoprogenitor cells. By day 5, chondrocytes usually are recognizable, and osteoblasts can be seen by posttransplantation day 10. Host blood vessels quickly infiltrate the graft through existing Haversian and Volkmann's canals and bring with them the osteoclasts that resorb the surfaces of the graft. Both intramembranous and endochondral bone formations usually occur on graft surfaces. Osteoconduction continues in large cortical or cancellous grafts for many years and ultimately results in the resorption of the original graft tissue and replacement with new host bone [6]. Biomechanical forces such as weight bearing will result remodeling. Thus, graft incorporation is a dynamic interplay of the biologic function, the graft environment, and the mechanical interactions between the host and graft [2].

Autografts generally are more rapidly and completely integrated into the host than allografts. Autologous bone graft is still considered to be the golden standard of bone grafting materials although patients must undergo the pain and possible complications associated with the harvesting procedure. Allogeneic and xenogeneic bone grafts carry with them a theoretical risk of disease transmission and increased cost. Since synthetic alloplastic materials can be precisely controlled for their physical and biological properties and are not constrained by limitations of additional surgical procedures for their fabrication, they are considered to be the most promising bone grafting materials.

7.2 Autograft and Allograft

Ideal bone graft substitutes should contain all three prerequisites for new bone formation. Those are osteoconductive matrix to provide physical support and reparative process framework that also function as synthetic extracellular matrix, osteoinductive factors to induce bone formation, and osteogenic stem cells that are capable to differentiate into bone-forming cells. In view of that, autograft is considered a golden standard. It was first used (to trace back from the literature) in the early 1800s. After drilling holes to release pressure in the skull, Walther [9] repaired the defect by refilling the hole with the original bone plug. The repair resulted in good healing and informally began the practice of autografting [10]. Since that, more reports on autografting emerged [11]. One of the most primary reasons for the success of autografts is its osteoinductive ability due to the presence of blood, factors, and proteins within the graft that stimulate and facilitate healing [10]. Although autografts provide the best replacement tissue to a defect site, the harvesting procedure requires an additional surgery in the donor site, which can result in complications, most commonly pain and risk infection. It was reported that the donor site morbidity occurs in approximately 20% of all cases [12, 13].

To overcome the problems in autografting, allograft began to be used as the substitute for autografts in large defect sites. Based on the literature studies by Laurencin and Khan [10], allograft use began to be reported in the late 1800s when Macewen reported on the implantation of tibial graft from one child to another [14, 15]. Meanwhile, bone banks were established in the beginning of the twentieth century when Bauer refrigerated bone samples for 3 weeks and then implanted them in a dog [10]. Bauer prepared bone storage at that time by chilling and heating, but it was soon found out that boiling the bone samples rendered them inferior to autografts because the endogenous proteins and factors undoubtedly destroyed during heating [16]. During the World War II, the big leap forward came when new methods for bone storage were studied including freezing, freeze-drying, deproteinating, irradiating, autoclaving, demineralizing, and chemically treating the harvested bone. The Naval projects [15] brought understanding that fresh allograft tissue declined sharply in orthopedic procedures. Although allografts carry with them the risk for disease transmission and adverse immunological reaction, donor screening and tissue processing methodologies have reduced the risk of allografts; thus it has become a more attractive alternative for autografts.

Allograft bone may be mineralized or demineralized. The properties of both mineralized and demineralized may be significantly affected by different processing and sterilization techniques. Mineralized allograft is available in several forms such as fresh, frozen, and freeze-dried. Because of its processing, sterilization, and preservation techniques, mineralized allograft's osteoinductivity, osteoconductivity, immunogenicity, mechanical strength, and potential for disease transmission may differ between similar types of allografts, depending on the procedures employed in their production [16]. Most allografts are either frozen or freeze-dried. Frozen allografts are maintained at temperatures below −60 °C to diminish degradation by enzymes, affording decrease immunogenicity [17]. Freeze-drying (also called lyophilization) involves the removal of water from the frozen tissue, after which the tissues are vacuum packed and stored at room temperature for up to 5 years [18]. Freeze-drying methods decrease antigenicity, even further, and may reduce the limited osteoinductive properties [16, 17]. However, freeze-drying method makes allograft more brittle that may be associated with the damage in the bone matrix, specifically micro cracks along the collagen fiber [19]. According to the previous studies, the properties of the freeze-dried allografts can be partially regained by rehydrating procedure prior to the grafting procedure [20].

For demineralized allografts, acid demineralization leaves behind an allograft composite of non-collagenous protein, bone growth factors, and collagen. It is known as DBM (demineralized bone matrix). Low molecular weight glycoproteins such as BMPs are said to be the most important factors in DBM; however it also contains other important factors: osteopontin, osteocalcin, and osteonectin [10, 21, 22]. There have been no adverse effects associated with the use of DBM because demineralization process reduces the risk of disease transmission to essentially zero; however processing chemicals and additives may be potentially toxic if very large dose of DBM is used. Thus, for clinical applications of DBM, manufacturers should be required to disclose all additives and chemicals used.

It is vitally important to dental implantologist, oral surgeons, or clinicians to understand that variations in processing may lead to significant differences in efficacy of the DBM. The manufacturers may not necessarily give this information. Several forms of processing are known to affect the biological properties or bone-forming capacity of DBM; some may be beneficial, while others have negative effects. Processing steps that are known to have a negative effect on osteoinduction include preprocessing storage of >24 h at 25 °C or higher, pulverization that yields particle sizes <75 mm, certain chelating agents such as EDTA, various acid-alcohol preparations, alternatives decalcifying solutions, excessive heat during processing, multiple freeze-thaw cycles, and tissue fixatives [10]. Methods that have beneficial effects on osteoinduction include decalcification with HCl (0.6 N); defatting with chloroform and ethanol, detergent rinsing; alcohol treatment; antibiotics such as oxytetracycline, erythromycin, and merthiolate; and lyophilization [10]. Exposure of DBM to terminally sterilization using ethylene oxide gas results in marked reduction of its osteoinductivity due to destruction of BMPs and other osteoinductive factors, and it is known to be dose-dependent [23]. Other methods of sterilization such as the use of ethanol may have less potential to reduce osteoinductive properties of DBM [24, 25]. Therefore, it is imperative for clinicians to understand and be aware how processing factors influence the efficacy of a particular DBM product for a particular clinical situation.

Another issue on the use of chemicals and additives should be clearly understood by clinicians. It is vital that the safety profile of all is known and clearly given by all manufacturers. It is suggested that the following information should be mandatory provided by DBM manufacturers. Those are type and quantity of additives, including residual of processing chemicals; safety profile of each additives; viral inactivation data; and activity data. Issues on the forms and fusion rate are also important. Commercially available DBM exists in flowable form (gel), pliable forms that maintain dimensional integrity (flex), and moldable forms that maintain cohesiveness (putty). Pliable and moldable forms are fiber based, and flowable forms are particle based. The fibrous structures significantly have greater osteoconductivity compared to gel formulation [10].

7.3 Synthetically Derived Bone Grafting

So far autografts remain the gold standard for bone graft procedures, and hence it is the most widely used. It is osteogenic and the risk of infection is minimal. However, there is significant patient morbidity associated with it, especially in the elderly and critical defects. Thus, allografts are alternative to autografts. However, by the rise of HIV- and hepatitis-infected cases in recent years, allografts carry with them increased risk of infection. Although sterilization techniques have been applied, but the sterilization techniques effect on the structural properties, such as reduced in toughness and detrimental effects on collagen. Given the limitations of autografts and allografts, there have been efforts for decades to find suitable synthetic bone graft materials.

7.3.1 Ceramics

Ceramics are highly crystalline structures formed by heating nonmetallic mineral salts to high temperatures in a process known as sintering, in the form of granules, porous blocks, and cements. Many ceramics are known to be biocompatible and have already been used in clinics for various applications. The temperature at which porous ceramics are sintered can affect biological response due to alteration of chemical and topographical surfaces of the materials [26]. Crystallinity also influences cell and tissue response by affecting the adsorption of serum components to the surface and the ability of cells to attach, proliferate, and differentiate [27]. Morphological characteristics and granule size can also affect bone ingrowth [28]. Thus, ceramics morphology, crystallinity, and chemical as well as topographical surfaces can be modified to improve tissue responses, such as enhancement of cell attachment by fibronectin and laminin treatment of the ceramics surface.

According to Tanaka and Yamashita [29], ceramics are generally classified from their chemical compositions into two groups: calcium phosphate (CP) and others, including yttria (Y_2O_3)-stabilized tetragonal zirconia (ZrO_2) (Y-TZP), alumina (Al_2O_3), and some silicate and phosphate families of glasses and crystallized glasses (glass-ceramics), as depicted in Table 7.3. The most clinically used ceramics of CP groups are hydroxyapatite ($Ca_5(PO_4)_3OH$, HA) and β-tricalcium phosphate ($Ca_3(PO_4)_3$, β-TCP) because of their analogous inorganic components with hard tissues of vertebrates. Use of Y-TZP and alumina is due to their excellent mechanical strength and toughness. The glasses and crystallized glasses in the SiO_2-P_2O_5-CaO-Na_2O system are classified as bioactive glasses and bioactive glass-ceramics, known as bioactive and resorbable ceramics.

7.3.1.1 Hydroxyapatite

Among several bioceramics available in the clinics, hydroxyapatite is one of the families of orthophosphate molecules and considered as the most biologically compatible substances used as bone graft substitute material. Hydroxyapatite (HA) is the dominant inorganic component of the hard tissues of the human body. Hydroxyapatite is soluble in acidic solution, insoluble in alkaline solution, and slightly soluble in distilled water. Hydroxyapatite has been used in particulate or granule forms and porous blocks. The HA stoichiometric chemical formula is $Ca_{10}(PO_4)_6(OH)_2$ and shares similarities with the mineral phase of the bone. However, synthetic HA and bone apatite are very different. The difference is because most of HA are produced by sintering in high temperatures; thus the process results in highly crystalline HA which is difficult to be resorbed during the remodeling process of the bone.

Meanwhile, bone apatite is highly carbonated and nonstoichiometric and exists as very small platelike crystals in three-dimensional matrix with dynamic arrangements, while synthetic HA tend to be homogenous in composition with larger and more perfect crystal. Bone apatite contains numerous ion substitutions. Table 7.4 lists the compositions of enamel, dentin, and bone apatite [30]. As shown in Table 7.4, the biological apatite is composed of impurity ions such as carbonate, sodium, magnesium, etc. Carbonate is one of the most abundant impurity ions, and its content is about a weight of 4–8%. The incorporation of carbonate into HA caused an increase in solubility, a decrease in crystallinity, a change in crystal morphology, and an enhancement of chemical reactivity owing to the weak bonding. Bone apatite is actually more soluble in vivo than HA and increases the local

Table 7.3 Composition and shapes of the various bioceramics

Category	Materials and compositions	Shapes
Calcium phosphate (CP) group	*Hydroxyapatite* (HAp or HA) $Ca_5(PO_4)_3OH$	Sintered body (dense and porous) Powder Coating Composite Fiber
	β-Tricalcium phosphate (β-TCP) $Ca_3(PO_4)_2$	Sintered body (dense and porous) Powder
	Dicalcium phosphate anhydrate (monetite, DCPD, or DCPA) $CaHPO_4$	Powder
	Dicalcium phosphate dihydrate (brushite, DCP2, or DCPD) $CaHPO_42H_2O$	Powder
	Calcium pyrophosphate (CPP) $Ca_2P_2O_7$	Powder
	α-Tricalcium phosphate (α-TCP) $Ca_3(PO_4)_2$	Powder
	Tetracalcium phosphate (TeCP) $Ca_4(PO_4)_2O$	Powder
	Octacalcium phosphate (OCP) $Ca_8H_2(PO_4)_65H_2O$	Powder
	Amorphous calcium phosphate (ACP) $Ca_3(PO_4)_2nH_2O$	Powder
Others	*Yttria-stabilized tetragonal zirconia* (Y-TZP) Y_2O_3-ZrO_2	Sintered body (dense)
	Aluminum oxide (Alumina) Al_2O_3	Sintered body (dense)
	Titanium oxide (Titania) TiO_2	Sintered body (dense)
	Silicon nitride Si_3N_4	Sintered body (dense)
	Silicon carbide SiC	Sintered body (dense)
	Carbon C	Fiber
	Bioactive glasses system	
	SiO_2-P_2O_5-Na_2O-CaO	Bulk
	SiO_2-P_2O_5-Na_2O-K_2O-CaO-MgO	Bulk
	SiO_2-P_2O_5-CaO-Al_2O_3	Bulk
	Bioactive glasses ceramics system	
	SiO_2-P_2O_5-CaO-MgO (A-W)	Bulk
	SiO_2-P_2O_5-Na_2O-K_2O-CaO-MgO (Ceravital)	Fiber

concentration of calcium and phosphate ions that are necessary for new bone formation. Thus in recent years, there are a lot of research that have shifted the use of HA into the biologically identical bone apatite which is carbonate hydroxyapatite (CHA), hydroxyapatite with carbonate ion substitutions.

Table 7.4 Hard tissue components of the human adult

	Enamel	Dentin	Bone
Ca^{2+}	36.5	35.1	34.8
PO_4 as P	17.7	16.9	15.2
Ca/P molar ratio	1.63	1.61	1.71
Na^+	0.5	0.6	0.9
Mg^{2+}	0.44	1.23	0.72
K^+	0.08	0.05	0.03
CO_3^{2-}	3.50	5.6	7.4
F^-	0.01	0.06	0.03
Cl^-	0.30	0.01	0.13
$P_2O_7^{4-}$	0.022	0.10	0.07
Total inorganic	97.0	70.0	65.0
Absorbed H_2O	1.5	10.0	10.0

The fingerprint of CHA is the substitution of carbonate ions for OH site and PO_4 site, which are defined as A-type and B-type, respectively. The main component of the biological apatite is B-type carbonate apatite. Solubility of CHA increases with carbon contents in both types. This leads to increased possibility of resorbability compared with pure HA. Ellies et al. [31] made a quantitative assessment of in vivo tissue biocompatibility of synthetic sintered carbonate apatite and found that increase in new bone formation corresponds to the increased in carbonate contents.

7.3.1.2 Coral-Derived Products

Coralline bone graft is derived from marine coral. Natural corals have a highly porous exoskeleton similar to the cancellous bone. Coral contains aragonite type of $CaCO_3$. It has been used in its natural mineral form of calcium carbonate, but to some extent it is also converted into calcium hydroxyapatite. This material is already used for bone grafting since 1970 because of its good osteoconduction, bioresorbability, biocompatibility, and biodegradation [32, 33]. The marine coral is made of aragonite-type calcium carbonate (97%), shows morphologically a porous microstructure, and is chemically quite similar to bone mineral. Coral shows a good tissue response and is completely resorbed in the body. Moreover, coral (aragonite or calcite forms of calcium carbonate or $CaCO_3$) is one of the limited numbers of materials that can form a chemical bond with the bone and soft tissues in vivo. Coral-derived bone graft substitutes are available in granular and block form. Depending on the type of material, the pore sizes may vary. The advantage of the coral-derived materials is that the pores are interconnected so that the bone can grow throughout the interstices of the implants.

Combes and coworkers [34] demonstrated the application of 100% calcium carbonate as a good bone cement candidate due to the re-crystallization of the initial metastable phases of the cement, in which $CaCO_3$ reacts with water, forms a calcium phosphate layer in the presence of phosphate ions, and acts as a template to facilitate apatite crystal formation and growth. Such a cement can be prepared by simply mixing water with $CaCO_3$ powder. After implantation, the cement will release calcium and carbonate ions, which subsequently can be incorporated into the apatite structure of the surrounding bone tissue. The released calcium ions inhibit the activity of osteoclasts and shift the bone balance toward formation [35]. Meanwhile, the carbonate ions released from $CaCO_3$ can substitute phosphates and or hydroxide ions in the structure of bone apatite.

7.3.1.3 Tricalcium Phosphate

The chemical formula of tricalcium phosphate (TCP) is $Ca_3(PO_4)_2$, which has four polymorphs: α, β, γ, and super-α. The γ polymorph is a high-pressure phase, and super-α polymorph is observed at temperatures above 1500 °C. The α-polymorph can set with simple two-way step reactions to form calcium-deficient hydroxyapatite (CDHA). When mixed with water, dissolution of TCP to supply Ca^{2+} and PO_4^{3-} and precipitation into CDHA will lead to the formation of needlelike crystals of apatite which interlock each other to form a set mass [36] in the following reaction:

$$3Ca_3(PO_4)_2 + H_2O \rightarrow 9Ca^{2+} + 6PO_4^{3-} + H_2O \text{ as dissolution} \quad (7.1)$$

$$9Ca^{2+} + 6PO_4^{3-} + H_2O \rightarrow Ca_9HPO_4(PO_4)_5(OH) \text{ as precipitation} \quad (7.2)$$

Unfortunately, setting time of α-TCP is too long if free from additives. This long setting time prevents its clinical use. Therefore, a chelating agent such as succinic acid or citric acid is employed to shorten the initial setting reaction, but it prevents compositional transformation to apatite.

In general TCP is less crystalline than hydroxyapatite and, therefore, more soluble. Bone graft that contains TCP is biocompatible and osteoconductive, but because of its relative solubility, it is used in the situation where structural support is less important. Both α- and β-TCP are high-temperature TCP with similar composition to amorphous calcium phosphate but with increased crystallinity. The difference is their crystal structures according to the order of temperature where α-TCP is the stable phase above 1125 °C, whereas β-TCP is below 1125 °C. The α-TCP is more soluble than β-TCP and reported to be more easily degraded in vivo. Compared to β-TCP, α-TCP has a lower density and a higher free energy of formation and is therefore expected to be more reactive [37]. Both α- and β-TCP are available in block, granule, or powder form.

7.3.1.4 Biphasic Calcium Phosphate

For β-TCP, commercially available one is also found in the form of biphasic calcium phosphate (BCP), a composite of hydroxyapatite and β-TCP. It is rapidly degradable compared to hydroxyapatite only. Because BCP is biphasic of hydroxyapatite and β-TCP, its chemical properties are determined by the ratio of HA to β-TCP. Several attempts are made to prepare BCP with different ratios of hydroxyapatite and β-TCP; one of them is by preparing HA and β-TCP independently, mixed mechanically, and followed by sintering procedure at proper temperatures. For more homogenous one, other methods are employed by transformation of calcium-deficient apatite into BCP. The transformation of calcium-deficient apatite into BCP can be prepared from dicalcium phosphate anhydrate (DCPA), dicalcium phosphate dihydrate (DCPD), α- or β-TCP, and octacalcium phosphate.

The bioactivity of the BCP can be obtained by an increase in calcium and phosphate concentration in local microenvironment by partial dissolution of BCP, formation of carbonate apatite from biological fluid, association of carbonate apatite crystals with an organic matrix, and incorporation of microcrystals with the collagenous matrix in the newly formed bone [38].

7.3.1.5 Calcium Phosphate Cement

Brown and Chow were the first to invent calcium phosphate cement that could be constituted at room temperature from calcium phosphate powder and water in 1985 [10, 39]. Calcium phosphate cements form on mixing a range of calcium phosphates with an aqueous solution, resulting in dissolution of calcium followed by a precipitation reaction in which calcium phosphate crystals grow and cement become rigid. Calcium phosphate is biocompatible and relevant to human hard tissue because the dominant inorganic component of human hard tissue is apatite, one of the types of calcium phosphate. Table 7.5 describes calcium orthophosphate or calcium phosphate and their solubility product constant [38].

Calcium phosphate can be categorized into two: apatite and brushite. Apatite cements form hydroxyapatite as an end product, although some have carbonate present and form carbonate apatite. Carbonate apatite is more degradable than hydroxyapatite, but both are considered to degrade slowly. Brushite cements degrade to form dicalcium phosphate dihydrate (DCPD) and are more degradable than apatite cements. Brushite can gradually transform to apatite in physiological conditions. Table 7.6 shows the categorization of the calcium phosphate cements.

Calcium phosphate cements have been used as carriers for growth factors, antibiotics, and bone morphogenetic factors. The compressive strength is strong but the tensile strength is low. Thus, calcium phosphate cements are suitable for treatment of fractures and defects that are not weight bearing. Calcium phosphate cements are generally unsuitable for diaphyseal fractures.

Table 7.5 Calcium phosphate and their solubility product constant

Compound	Abbreviation	Chemical formula	Ca/P	Log (Ksp)
Monocalcium phosphate monohydrate	MCPM	$Ca(H_2PO_4)_2.H_2O$	0.5	Highly soluble
Monocalcium phosphate anhydrous	MCPA	$Ca(H_2PO_4)_2$	0.5	Highly soluble
Dicalcium phosphate dihydrate	DCPD	$CaHPO_4.2H_2O$	1.0	6.59
Dicalcium phosphate anhydrate	DCPA	$CaHPO_4$	1.0	6.90
Octacalcium phosphate	OCP	$Ca_8H_2(PO_4)_6.5H_2O$	1.33	96.6
α-Tricalcium phosphate	α-TCP	$Ca_3(PO_4)_2$	1.5	
β-Tricalcium phosphate	β-TCP	$Ca_3(PO_4)_2$	1.5	28.9
Hydroxyapatite	HA	$Ca_{10}(PO_4)_6(OH)_2$	1.67	116.8
Fluorapatite	FA	$Ca_{10}(PO_4)_6F_2$	1.67	121
Tetracalcium phosphate	TTCP	$Ca_4(PO_4)_2O$	2.0	38–44

Table 7.6 Properties of calcium phosphate cements

	Apatite cement	Brushite cement
End product	Hydroxyapatite (HA) or carbonate apatite (CHA)	Dicalcium phosphate dihydrate (DCPD)
Degradability	Degrade slowly, faster in carbonate apatite	More degradable than apatite cements Resorbed more quickly, by dissolution as well as osteoclast resorption
Mechanical properties	Vary between cements, depend on the composition Increase overtime in vivo	Vary between cements, depend on the composition Decrease rapidly in vivo but increase with the increased healing bone
Biocompatibility	Biocompatible, few inflammatory reactions have been reported	Biocompatible, inflammatory reactions have been reported

7.3.2 Bioactive Glasses

Bioactive glasses were discovered by Hench and coworkers in 1969. Currently there are various bioactive glasses and bioactive glass-ceramics available for clinical applications. Table 7.7 shows various compositions of bioactive glasses and glass-ceramics available for clinical applications [40]. The family of bioactive glasses contains SiO_2, Na_2O, CaO, and P_2O_5 in specific proportions. The glasses differ from traditional soda-lime-silica glasses in three compositional features as follows: less than 60 mol% SiO_2, high Na_2O, and CaO contents, with high CaO/P_2O_5 ratio. These features make glass surface highly reactive when it is exposed to an aqueous medium.

Bioactive glasses are also ceramics, or it is usually considered as surface-reactive ceramics. Bioactive glasses are formed by melting or sol-gel techniques. They are available in sintered porous bulk or particulate form. The surface of the bioactive glasses is an important part of the glasses because it takes part in a reaction with host tissue on implantation. The surface of the glass will be dissolved and release mineral ions. This leads to the formation of a biologically active, carbonated apatite layer that provides the bonding interface with tissues. This adherent interface with tissues resists substantial mechanical forces. In many cases, the interfacial strength of adhesion is equivalent to or greater than the cohesive strength of the implant material or the tissue bonded to the bioactive implant.

A study done by El-ghannam and coworkers [41] shows that initial reaction of some bioactive glasses causes a local increase in pH; thus alkalinization is beneficial to cell activity and hydroxyapatite production. By the initial reaction on the surface of the bioactive glasses, calcium phosphate layer is formed, and the layer is thought to enhance protein adsorption on the surface of the implant. The process is then involved in the surface reaction with the host bone.

In other references, El-ghannam and coworkers [42] found that surface-treated bioglass has been shown to adsorb fibronectin more selectively than do hydroxyapatite ceramics. The presence of both the calcium phosphate layer and serum proteins has been shown to influence the behavior of osteoblast on the surface of materials.

Table 7.7 Properties of calcium phosphate cements [40]

Component	Glass and glass-ceramics									
	45S5 Bioglass	45S5F Bioglass	45S5.4F Bioglass	40S5B5 Bioglass	52S4.6 Bioglass	55S4.3 Bioglass	KGC Ceravital	KGS Ceravital	KGy213 Ceravital	AW-GC
SiO_2	45	45	45	40	52	55	46.2	46	38	34.2
P_2O_5	6	6	6	6	6	6				16.3
CaO	24.5	12.25	14.7	24.5	21	19.5	20.2	33	31	44.9
$Ca(PO_3)_2$							25.5	16	13.5	
CaF_2		12.25	9.8							0.5
MgO							2.9			4.6
MgF_2										
Na_2O	24.5	24.5	24.5	24.5	21	19.5	4.8	5	4	
K_2O										
Al_2O_3									7	
B_2O_3				5						
Ta_2O_5/TiO_2									6.5	

Although some bioactive glass formulation are brittle and may form particular debris contributing to the release of inflammatory cytokines, bioactive glasses are biocompatible and in many clinical situation are as effective as hydroxyapatite or autologous bone graft.

7.3.3 Calcium Sulfate

Calcium sulfate (CS), also known as plaster of Paris (POP), has been used in clinic for many years to treat skeletal defects, either alone or in combination with other bone graft materials [43–46]. Calcium sulfate cement is one of the oldest and sturdiest building materials on earth. It is a gypsum product that has been used for at least 5000 years. It is safe, rapidly resorbing material that has been used for bone filling applications for more than 100 years. The use of POP is based on its advantages, which includes the ability to self-setting and a well-tolerated biological response without eliciting a severe inflammatory response. When hemihydrate is mixed with water, dihydrate is formed. This property makes it possible for POP to set in situ when it is applied into a bone defect. Figure 7.1 shows diagrammatical description on how CS or POP or gypsum sets. The setting mechanism of the CS is as follows:

$$CaSO_4 \cdot 0.5H_2O + 1.5H_2O \rightarrow CaSO_4 \cdot 2H_2O + Q \tag{7.3}$$

However, POP has a major setback as it is rapidly resorbed in vivo and consequently unable to provide a long-term three-dimensional framework to support osteoconduction [47, 48]. To overcome this problem of fast degradation, medical-grade POP has been mixed with other bone graft materials such as β-tricalcium

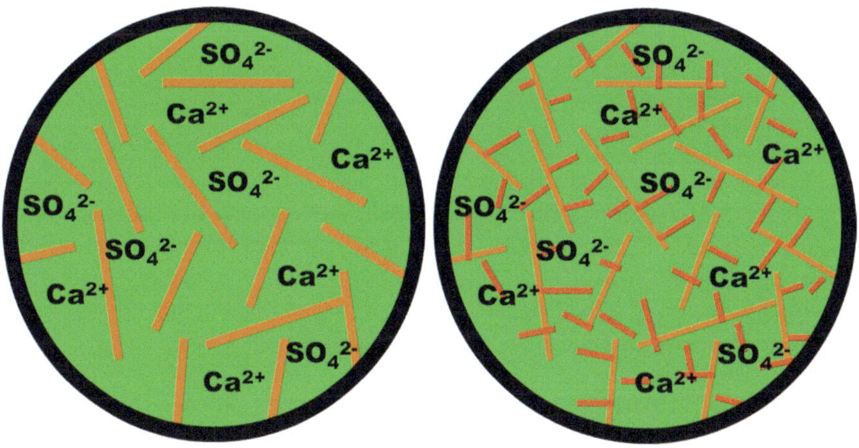

Fig. 7.1 Calcium sulfate (CS) or plaster of Paris (POP) or gypsum has ability to set (free molding). This is because of the large solubility (0.82 g/100 mL) of CS hemihydrate ($CaSO_4 \cdot 0.5H_2O$). When CS hemihydrate reacts with water, dehydrate is formed (low solubility (0.20 g/100 mL) of $CaSO_4 \cdot 2H_2O$)

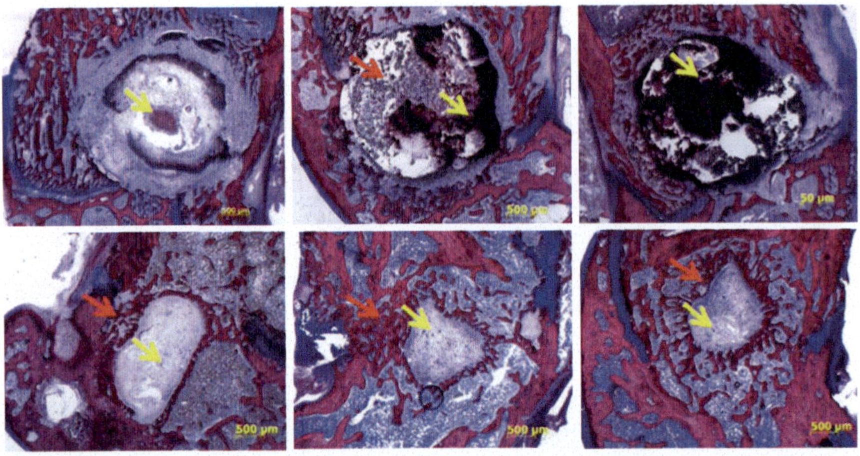

Fig. 7.2 Efforts have been being extensively done to fasten bone formation by combining CS with other materials. After the combination of CS with $CaCO_3$, the degradation rate of the materials is considered ideal for a bone substitute materials in terms of its capability to maintain space in bone defect area

phosphate, freeze-dried demineralized bone graft, and calcium phosphate. Dewi and co-workers [49–51] have been doing efforts to enhance bone formation in POP implantation to overcome problems related to fast degradability of POP. Figure 7.2 shows the result of the works [50]. When POP was mixed with $CaCO_3$ or hydrogel $CaCO_3$, faster bone formation was achieved, but the mechanical strength of the POP composite decreased significantly. Although the efforts have been being continued to improve properties of CS or POP as bone substitute [52], the use of CS alone is suggested in contained nonstructural defects or combined with fixation and other materials to enhance bone formation.

7.3.4 Polymers

Polymers are used in a variety of surgical applications. There are two kinds of polymers used in various surgical applications, non-resorbable and resorbable or biodegradable polymers. Non-resorbable polymers include ultrahigh molecular weight such as polyethylene (usually used as a bearing surface) and polymethyl methacrylate (usually used as acrylic cement for implant fixation and defect filling). Non-resorbable materials are not intended to be replaced with a bone, but they may interface with bone tissue.

Meanwhile, biodegradable polymers have several different applications. Bioresorbable polymers are used early for suture materials and internal fixation devices, such as polydioxanone and polyglicolide to avoid the need for removal. Recently, biodegradable polymers have expanded to be used as scaffold in tissue engineering in various forms such as porous membrane, porous blocks, and microsphere.

They are also developed as carrier materials for cells and growth factors, including other proteins. As a carrier material, biodegradable polymer is allowed to introduce osteogenic factors locally while providing a framework for ingrowth of new bone formation.

Most biodegradable polymers used as a scaffold in bone tissue engineering belong to polyhydroxy acid family [10] and include poly(L-lactide) and poly(D-L-lactide) or PLA, polyglicolide (PGA), and copolymers based on PLA and PGA. Other polymers are also in the pipeline for the development and studied extensively such as poly(propylene fumarate) (PPF), polycaprolactone, polysaccharides, etc. Polymer degradation, e.g., in polyhydroxy acid, results CO_2 and water, which are completely eliminated from the body. As a consequence of the hydrolysis process during degradation, the release of acidic products cannot be avoided, which in turn corresponds to the fall of local pH. As a result of hydrolysis process during polymer degradation, local inflammatory reactions have been reported, leading to the questions on the biocompatibility of polymer to be used as bone substitutes.

7.3.5 Composites

To counteract acidic loading during polymer degradation, basic salts or calcium compounds such as hydroxyapatite or tricalcium phosphate are added into polymers [53, 54]. This is because calcium compounds such as hydroxyapatite or tricalcium phosphate increase local pH during their decomposition processes. Beside buffering capabilities of calcium compounds such as hydroxyapatite or tricalcium phosphate, the incorporation of ceramics or calcium phosphate compounds into polymers allows the formation of composites that can be specifically designed to have predictable biomechanical properties and resorption rate. Some have been commercialized such as the combination of gelatin with CHA [55]. Figure 7.3 shows microstructure of the commercially available CHA composite.

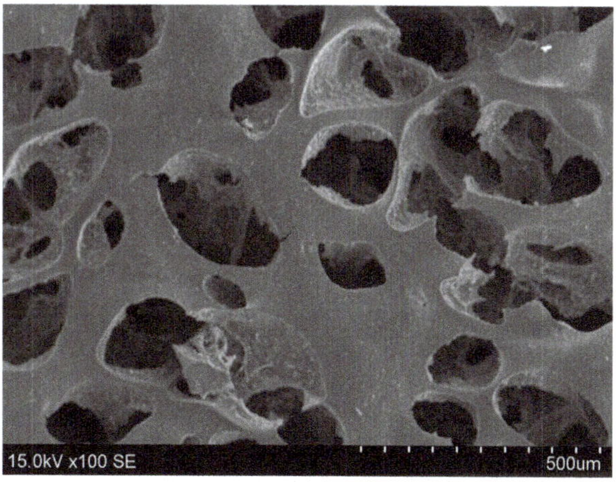

Fig. 7.3 Microstructure of CHA composite commercially available and known as Gama-CHA

Simultaneously, a lot of studies have been being done extensively to investigate factors influencing chemical, physical, and biomechanical properties of polymers and their composites. The factors include the chemical structure, morphology, composition, ratio of components, and addition of low molecular weight components, including the fabrication or synthesis techniques and possibilities for various applications [56–58].

7.4 Current Perspective and Future Directions

Despite the decades of biomaterial research, synthetic bone substituting materials are still largely inferior to auto- or allografts as the gold standard in orthopedics and dental surgery. The clinical success of the current generation of bone substituting materials is disappointingly limited since they lack high functionality of bone tissue in terms of biological and mechanical properties [59, 60].

When a tissue is severely damaged or lost, not only large numbers of functional cells but also the matrix in tissue, generally called extracellular matrix (ECM), are lost. It has been a critical issue and a key challenge in the regenerative area on how to ideally replace lost tissue. For this, the same natural healthy tissue or autograft is still considered to be the gold standard of grafting materials, but patients must undergo the pain and possible complication associated with the harvesting procedure. Allogeneic and xenogeneic grafts carry with them a theoretical risk of disease transmission and increased cost. This situation has led to the concept of engineering or regenerating new tissue.

A new therapeutic strategy, with its objective is to induce the regeneration and repair of defective tissues based on natural healing potential of the tissues, which is known as regenerative medical therapy has become an alternative for future challenges in medicine and dental implantology. Providing cells with an in vivo local environment which enables them to proliferate and differentiate efficiently which results to cell-induced tissue regeneration is the strategy in successful regenerative medical therapy. The previous mentioned concept is actually the basic of tissue engineering that was originally introduced by Langer and Vacanti [61, 62]. In general, tissue engineering is the field of functional restoration of structure and physiology for damaged or lost tissue. The three ingredients for tissue engineering are signals for morphogenesis, stem cells responding to the morphogens, and a scaffold to represent extracellular matrix.

In 1997, media all over the world were aroused by a BBC documentary, Tomorrow's World, showing what is known as Vacanti mouse which is adopted from an article by Cao and coworkers [63]. Since that, the term tissue engineering was no longer familiar to only limited number of scientist working in the field, but it had become a well-known term to millions of individuals worldwide. Although the Vacanti experiment is truly exemplary for the discipline of tissue engineering, the news aroused in the media was not caused by the actual experiment but by spectacular picture of a nude mouse that had apparently grown a human ear on its back.

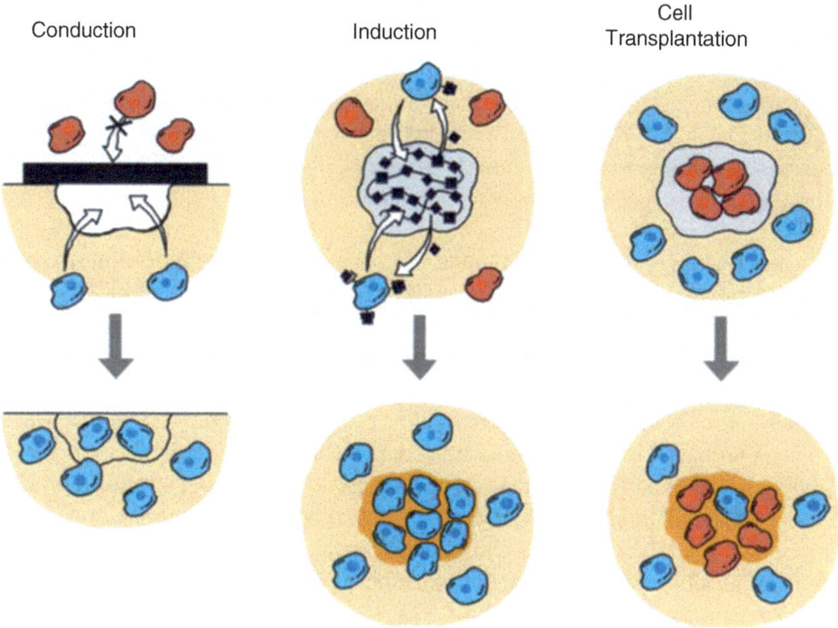

Fig. 7.4 Tissue engineering strategies as described by Alsberg et al. [64]. Figure is taken from Kaigler and Mooney [65]. The strategy has been being a hope and hype for future regenerative therapy, including in the area of dental implantology and maxillofacial surgery

The fundamental principles of tissue engineering involve two approaches: top-down and bottom-up approach. Examining and mimicking larger original structure is the basic concept of top-down approach, while assembling tissue from a cellular basis and scaling up into intact structure is of bottom-up approach. Based on a general description given by tissue engineering researchers, both approaches need conductive, inductive, and cell transplantation strategies, as described well by Kaigler and Mooney [64, 65] in Fig. 7.4.

The conductive strategy makes the use of a barrier membrane to exclude connective tissue cells that will interfere the regenerative process, while enabling the desired host cells to populate the regeneration site. The construct of the barrier membrane is also recognized to provide local environment for cells to promote proliferation and differentiation and function as instructive extracellular microenvironments for morphogenesis. It is composed of biological signal molecules, extracellular matrix (ECM) molecules, mechanical stress, and cell-to-cell interactions.

The inductive strategy uses biodegradable polymer scaffold as a vehicle to deliver growth factors and genes to the host site. The growth factors or genes can be released at a controlled rate based on the breakdown of the polymer. Previous researches have demonstrated that growth factors are efficiently used to regenerate various tissues. Several researches also deal with the attempt to use genes to promote blood vessel, soft tissues, bone, and cartilage regeneration. The cell transplantation strategy uses a similar vehicle as inductive strategy for delivery in order to transplant cells and partial tissues to the host site.

In view of the development in the regenerative strategy, nowadays stem cell treatments have been introduced extensively as well. Stem cells can be defined by two properties: the ability to make identical copies of cells (self-renewal) and the ability to form other cell types of the body (differentiation). For cell-induced tissue regeneration to succeed, it is often necessary to use stem cells. This is because ideally the cells used for tissue engineering should have the capacity to first proliferate and then differentiate. Unfortunately, the renewal capacity decreases by time. Thus, to learn how to control and regulate natural regeneration potential is a long-term goal in the context of tissue engineering. If there is in vitro manner that can be reproducibly controlled, cell differentiation and functional assembly can be guided.

Other future challenges are related to acidic condition caused by infections which have been problems in bone grafting procedures. Hospital-acquired bone infection, including in the maxillofacial area (even more specifically in tropical settings with high temperature/humidity), is a costly and critical health issue and the great difficulty to eradicate. Thus, it has led clinicians to consider the prevention of bone infection as an absolute necessity. Calcium phosphate apatites are best candidates for preparing biomaterials for bone repair. However, calcium phosphate compounds could act as propitious substrates for microbial proliferation. Despite the exponential industrial development of calcium phosphate compounds worldwide, there are no definite industrial strategies for conferring their inner antibacterial properties. Since the use of antibiotics is often problematic (bacterial resistance), other strategies have to be found, compared, and developed. In view of this, the development of ceramics such as apatite with inner antimicrobial properties is considered very strategic and important to overcome the problems in the near future [66].

References

1. Cha HS, Kim JW, Hwang JH, Ahn KM. Frequency of bone graft in implant surgery. Maxillofac Plast Reconstr. 2016;38(1):19. https://doi.org/10.1186/s40902-016-0064-2.
2. Goldberg FM, Akhavan S. Biology of bone grafts. In: Friedlander GE, Mankin HJ, Goldberg VM, editors. Bone grafts and bone graft substitutes, monograph series 32. American Academy of Orthopedic Surgeons: Rosemont, IL; 2006.
3. Burchardt H. Biology of bone transplantation. Orthop North Am. 1987;18:187–96.
4. Goldberg VM. Bone grafts and their substitutes: facts, fictions and failures. Orthopedics. 2001;24:875–6.
5. Basset C. Clinical implications of cell function in bone grafting. Clin Orthop. 1972;87:49–59.
6. Gray J, Elves M. Cearly osteogenesis in compact isografts: a quantitative study of contributions of different giant cells. Calcif Tissue Int. 1979;29:225–37.
7. Gray J, Elves M. Early osteogenesis in compact isografts: a quantitative study of contributions of the different graft cells. Clin Orthop. 1982;163:261.
8. Urist M. Bone transplantation. In: Urist M, editor. Fundamental and cinical bone phisiology. Philadelphia, PA: JB Lippincott; 1980.
9. Sanan A, Haines SJ. Repairing holes in the head: a history of cranioplasty. Neurosurgery. 1997;40:558–602.

10. Laurencin CT, Khan Y. Bone grafts and bone graft substitutes: a brief history. In: Laurencin CT, editor. Bone graft substitutes. American Academy of Orthopedic Surgeons: Rosemont, IL; 2003.
11. Meeder PJ, Eggers C. The history of autogenous bone grafting. Injury. 1994;25:A2–4.
12. Fleming JE, Cornell CN, Muschler GF. Bone cells and matrices in orthopedic tissue engineering. Orthop Clin North Am. 2000;31:357–74.
13. Perry CR. Bone repair techniques, bone graft, and bone graft substitutes. Clin Orthop Rel Res. 1999;360:71–86.
14. Czitrom AA, Gross AE. Allografts in orthopedic practice. Baltimore, MD: Williams and Wilkins; 1992.
15. Friedlaender GE, Mankin HJ, Sell KW. Osteochondral allograft biology, banking and clinical applications. Boston, MA: Little Brown and Co; 1983.
16. Boyce T, Edward J, Scarborough N. Allograft bone: the influence of processing on safety and performance. Orthop Clin North Am. 1999;20:571–80.
17. Gazdag AR, Lane JM, Glaser D, Forster RA. Alternatives to autogenous bone graft: Efficacy and indications. J Am Acad Orthop Surg. 1995;3:1–8.
18. Kagan RJ. Standards for tissue banking. Mc Lean: Vancouver, BC; 1998.
19. Voggenreiter G, Ascheri R, Blumel G. Effect of preservation and sterilization on cortical bone grafts: a scanning electron microscope study. Arch Orthop Trauma Surg. 1994;113:294–6.
20. Conrad EU, Ericksen DP, Tencer AF. The effects of freeze drying and rehydration on cancellous bone. Clin Orthop Rel Res. 1993;290:279–84.
21. Bauer TW, Muchsler GF. Bone graft materials: an overview of the basic science. Clin Orthop Rel Res. 2000;371:10–27.
22. Sandhu HS, Grewal HS, Parvataneni H. Bone grafting for spinal fusion. Orthop Clin North Am. 1999;30:685–98.
23. Doherty MJ, Mollan RAB, Wilson DJ. Effect of EOG sterilization on human demineralized bone. Biomaterials. 1993;15:994–8.
24. Dahners LE, Hoyle M. Chemical sterilization of bacterially contaminated bone without destruction of osteogenic potential. J Orthop Trauma. 1989;3:241–4.
25. Hallfeldt KKJ, Stutzle H, Puhlmann M, Kessler S, Schweiberer L. Sterilization of partially demineralized bone matrix: the effects of different sterilization techniques on osteogenic properties. J Surg Res. 1995;59:614–20.
26. Frayssinet P, Rouquet N, Fages J, Durant M, Vidalain PO, Bonel G. The influence of sintering temperature on the proliferation of fibroblastic cells in contact with HA bioceramics. J Biomed Mater Res. 1997;35:337–47.
27. Frank RM, Klewansky P, Hemmerle J, Tenenbaum H. Ultrastructure demonstration of the importance of crystal size of bioceramic powders implanted into human periodontal lesions. J Clin Periodontal. 1991;18:669–80.
28. Oonishi H, Hench LL, Wilson J, Sugihara F, Tsuji E, Kushitani S, Iwaki H. Comparative bone growth behavior in granules of bioceramic materials of various sizes. J Biomed Mater Res. 1999;44:31–43.
29. Tanaka Y, Yamashita K. Fabrication processes of bioceramics. In: Kokubo T, editor. Bioceramics and their clinical applications. Cambridge: Woodhead Publishing; 2008.
30. Le Geroz RZ. Calcium phosphate in oral biology and medicine. Monogr Oral Sci, vol. 15. Basel: Karger Publisher; 1991.
31. Ellies LG, Carter JM, Natiella JR, Featherstone JDB, Nelson DGA. Quantitative analysis of early in vivo tissue response to synthetic apatite implants. J Biomed Mater Res. 1988;22:137–48.
32. Chun Wu Y, Min Lee T, Hsun Chiu K, Yu Shaw S, Yu Yang C. A comparative study of the physical and mechanical properties of three natural corals based on the criteria for bone-tissue engineering scaffolds. J Mater Sci Mater Med. 2009;20:1273–80.
33. Cirotteau Y. Behavior of natural coral in a human osteoporotic bone. Eur J Orthop Surg Traumatol. 2001;11:149–60.

34. Combes C, Miao B, Bareille R, Rey C. Preparation, physical-chemical characterization and cytocompatibility of calcium carbonate cements. Biomaterials. 2006;27:1945–54.
35. Kameda T, Mano H, Yamada Y, Takai H, Amizuka N, Kobori M, Izumi N, Kawashima H, Ozawa H, Ikeda K, Kameda A, Hakeda Y, Kumegawa M. Calcium-sensing receptor in mature osteoclasts, which are bone-resorbing cells. Biochem Biphys Res Commun. 1998;245:419–22.
36. Tsuru K, Ruslin R, Maruta M, Matsuya S, Ishikawa K. Effects of the method of apatite seed crystals addition on setting reaction of α-tricalcium phosphate based apatite cement. J Mater Sci Mater Med. 2015;26(10):244–9.
37. Bohner M, Merkle HP, Van Landuyt P, Trophardy G, Lemaitre J. Effect of several additives and their admixtures on the physico-chemical properties of a calcium phosphate cement. J Mater Sci Mater Med. 1996;7:457–63.
38. Ishikawa K, Matsuya S, Miyamoto Y, Kawate K. Bioceramics. In: Milne I, Ritchie RO, Karihaloo BL, editors. Comprehensive structural integrity. Michigan: Elsevier; 2003.
39. Brown W, Chow L. Dental restorative cement pastes, US patent no. 4518430; 1985.
40. Wang M. Bioactive materials and processing. In: Shi D, editor. Biomaterials and tissue engineering. Berlin: Springer; 2004.
41. El-ghannam A, Ducheyne P, Saphiro IM. Formation of surface reaction products of bioactive glass and their effects on the expression of the osteoblastic phenotype and the deposition of mineralized extracellular matrix. Biomaterials. 1997;18:295–303.
42. El-ghannam A, Ducheyne P, Saphiro IM. Effect of serum proteins on osteoblast adhesion to surface-modified bioactive glass and hydroxyapatite. J Orthop Res. 1999;17:340–5.
43. Iezzi G, Fiera E, Scarano A, Pecora G, Piatelli A. Histologic evaluation of provisional implant retrieved from man 7 months after placement in a sinus augmented with calcium sulfate: a case report. J Oral Implant. 2007;33(2):89–95.
44. Jamali A, Hilpert A, Debes J, Afshar P, Rahban S, Holmes R. Hydroxyapatite/calcium carbonate (HA/CC) vs. plaster of Paris: a histomorphometric and radiographic study in a rabbit tibial defect model. Calcif Tissue Int. 2002;1:172–8.
45. Mazor Z, Mamidwar S, Ricci JL, Tovar NM. Bone repair in periodontal defect using a composite of allograft and calcium sulfate (dentogen) and a calcium sulfate barrier. J Oral Implantol. 2011;37(2):287–92.
46. Orsini G, Ricci J, Scarano A, Pecora G, Petrone G, Iezzi G, Piatelli A. Bone-defect healing with calcium-sulfate particles and cement: an experimental study in rabbit. Int J Oral Maxillofac Implant. 2004;24:901–9.
47. Ricci JL, Alexander H, Nadkarni P, Hawkins M, Turner J, Rosenblum SF, Brezenoff L, De Leonardis D, Pecora G. Biological mechanism of calcium sulfate replacement by bone. In: Davies JE, editor. Bone engineering. Toronto, ON: Em Squared Inc; 2000.
48. Thomas MV, Puleo DA. Review calcium sulfate: properties and clinical application. J Biomed Mater Res Part B Appl Biomater. 2008;88B:597–610.
49. Dewi AH, Ana ID, Jansen JA. Calcium carbonate hydrogel construct with cynnamaldehyde incorporated to control inflammation during surgical procedure. J Biomed Mater Res Part A. 2016;104:768–74.
50. Dewi AH, Ana ID, Wolke JGC, Jansen JA. Behavior of plaster of Paris-calcium carbonate composite as bone substitute. A study in rats. J Biomed Mater Res A. 2013;101(8):2143–50.
51. Dewi AH, Ana ID, Wolke JGC, Jansen JA. Behavior of POP-calcium carbonate hydrogel as bone substitute with controlled release capability: a study in rat. 2015. J Biomed Mater Res A. 2015;103:3273–83.
52. Dewi AH, Ana ID, Jansen JA. Preparation of a calcium carbonate-based bone substitute with cinnamaldehyde crosslinking agent with potential anti-inflammatory properties. J Biomed Mater Res A. 2017;105(4):1055–62.
53. Agrawal CM, Athanasiou KA. Technique to control pH in vicinity of biodegrading PLA-PGA implants. J Biomed Mater Res A. 1997;38:105–14.
54. Thomson RC, Yaszemski MJ, Powears JM, Mikos AG. Hydroxyapatite fiber reinforced Poly (alpha-hydroxy ester) foams for bone regeneration. Biomaterials. 1998;19:1935–43.

55. Leeuwenburgh SCG, Ana ID, Jansen JA. Sodium citrate as an effective dispersant for the synthesis of inorganic-organic composites with a nanodispersed mineral phase. Acta Biomater. 2010;6(3):836–44.
56. Ardhani R, Hafiyyah OA, Setyaningsih AID. Preparation of carbonate apatite membrane as metronidazole delivery for periodontal application. KEM. 2016;696:250–8.
57. Patriati A, Ardhani R, Pranowo HD, Ana ID. Effect of freeze-thaw treatment to the properties of gelatin carbonated hydroxy apatite membrane for nerve regeneration scaffold. Key Eng Mater. 2016;696:129–44.
58. Sunarso S, Tsuru K, Ana ID, Ishikawa K. Effect of crosslinking to the mechanical properties of apatite gelatin hybrid for bone substitution purposes. Indo J Chem. 2011;11(3):267–72.
59. Kirkpatrick JC, Fuchs S, Peters K, Brochhausen C, Hermanns MI, Unger RE. Vision for regenerative medicine: interface between scientific fact and science fiction. Artif Organ. 2006;30:822–7.
60. Leeuwenburgh SCG, Jansen JA, Malda J, Dhert WA, Rouwkema J, Van Blitterswijk CA. Trends in biomaterials research: an analysis of the scientific programme of the World Biomaterials Congress. Biomaterials. 2008;29:3047–52.
61. Langer R, Vacanti JP. Tissue engineering. Science. 1993;260:920–6.
62. Vacanti JP, Langer R. Tissue engineering: the design and fabrication of living replacement devices for surgical reconstruction and transplantation. Lancet. 1999;354(Suppl.1):132–4.
63. Cao Y, Vacanti JP, Paige KT. Transplantation of chondrocytes utilizing a polymer-cell construct to produce tissue engineered cartilage in the shape of human ear. Plast Reconstr Surg. 1997;100:297–302.
64. Alsberg E, Hill E, Moonhey DJ. Craniofacial tissue engineering. Crit Rev Oral Biol Med. 2001;12(1):64–75.
65. Kaigler D, Mooney D. Tissue engineering's impact on dentistry. J Dent Educ. 2001;65(5):456–62.
66. Ana ID, Satria GAP, Dewi AH, Ardhani R. Bioceramics for clinical application in regenerative dentistry. Adv Exp Med Biol. 2018;1077:309–16.

Periimplantitis

8

Herbert Deppe

8.1 Introduction

Over the past decades, the placement of dental implants has become a routine procedure in the oral rehabilitation of fully and partially edentulous patients [1]. Due to the fact that the number of patients that undergo restorative therapy through dental implants increases, peri-implantitis is considered to be an increasing problem in dentistry.

At present, therapy of peri-implant infections is still a matter of debate. Several methods for implant neck instrumentation were characterized in vitro (stainless steel or titanium curettes; air polisher using glycine-based Perio or soft powders or erythritol powder; and an ultrasonic device using stainless steel or plastic-coated instruments) [2]. It was concluded that no significant differences were observed in the surface characteristics (except for stainless steel curettes) or bacterial colonization based on one-time instrumentation. Similarly, various methods and therapies were tested in vivo [3]. The authors have stated from a review that peri-implantitis lesions were most frequently induced in dogs and were found to have many clinical and histological features in common with naturally occurring lesions observed in humans. Moreover, cross-sectional studies on implant-treated subjects are rare, and only few of them provide data on the prevalence of peri-implant diseases. Due to the literature available, peri-implant mucositis occurred in 1–47% of the subjects, whereas peri-implantitis was identified in 19–65% of subjects (Leitlinie DGZMK). Derks and Tomasi [4] reported in a systematic review a weighted mean prevalence of peri-implantitis of 22% (95% confidence interval, 14–30%) with a positive relationship between prevalence and time in function of the implants. As one of the

H. Deppe (✉)
Department of Oral, Maxillofacial and Plastic Surgery, Technische Universität München, Munich, Germany
e-mail: herbert.deppe@tum.de

A. S. Budihardja, T. Mücke (eds.), *Bone Management in Dental Implantology*,
https://doi.org/10.1007/978-3-319-78951-4_8

difficulties, it was reported that heterogeneous diagnostic criteria are used to define peri-implant mucositis [5]. Differences in the definition of peri-implantitis have resulted in a wide range of reported prevalence values. Such differences include the use of different thresholds for bone loss, inflammatory parameters (BOP, PPD) and differences in the combination thereof [6]. Reviews have recognized seven case definitions for peri-implantitis based on the amount of bone loss occurring over time [4, 7, 8]. Recently, it was reported that a total of 13 definitions for peri-implantitis were available in the literature [5]. Although bleeding on probing was a consistently used parameter in the studies included in the systematic review, case definitions frequently applied other parameters (e.g. probing depth) resulting in inconsistent distinction between health and disease [1]. Therefore, the inter-rater agreement in the diagnosis of mucositis and peri-implantitis was assessed in a clinical study [9]. Interestingly, a complete agreement was obtained only in 52% of cases. Accordingly, the inter-rater agreement in the diagnosis of peri-implant disease was qualified as merely good, based in part on the unclear definition of peri-implantitis and mucositis.

Peri-implantitis lesions are larger and present with more aggressive features than lesions in periodontitis around teeth [10]. During 3 weeks of plaque accumulation, the median plaque index and gingival index increased significantly at both implants and teeth. However, over a 6-week experimental period, the crevicular fluid levels of MMP-8 were statistically significantly higher at implants compared with teeth [11]. In a 5-year follow-up study, the incidence of peri-implantitis in individuals with mucositis was determined. Without preventive maintenance during the study period, the incidence of peri-implantitis was 43.9% and with preventive maintenance 18.0% [12]. Untreated disease leads to spontaneous progression [13] and to loss of implants [14].

Recently, state of the art in diagnosis and treatment of peri-implant diseases was published by the German Society for Dental and Oral Medicine (DGZMK) [15] and Schwarz and coworkers [16]. This chapter is based on these publications.

8.2 Diagnosis of Peri-implant Diseases

8.2.1 Definition

Peri-implant diseases present in two forms—peri-implant mucositis and peri-implantitis [17]. Peri-implant mucositis and peri-implantitis are infectious diseases. Peri-implant mucositis describes an inflammatory lesion that resides in the mucosa, while peri-implantitis also affects the supporting bone [18] (Fig. 8.1).

8.2.2 Aetiology

It is clearly demonstrated in the literature that plaque accumulation results in peri-implant mucositis around osseointegrated dental implants [19]. The host response to biofilms does not differ substantially at teeth or implants [20]. Smoking has been

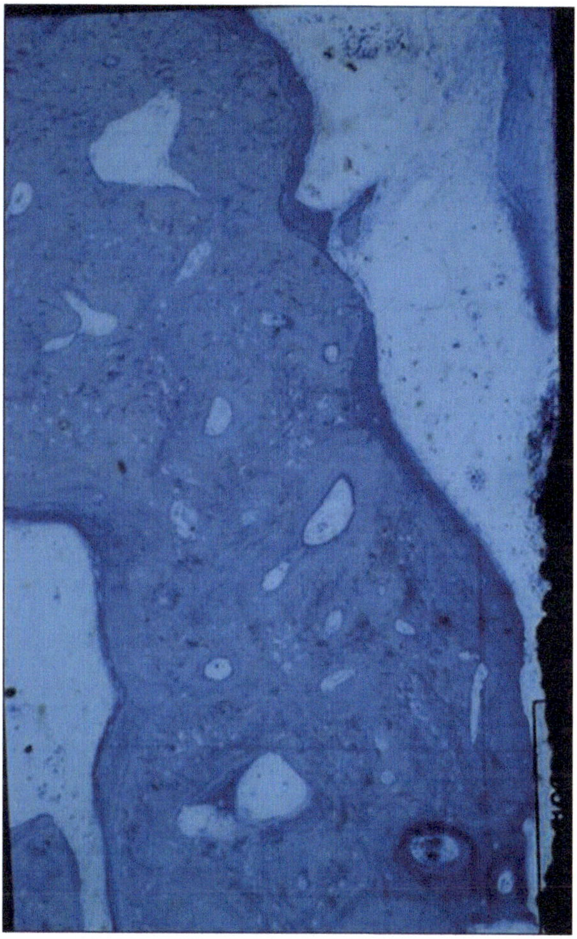

Fig. 8.1 Section of an implant with clinical signs of peri-implantitis. Bone loss is clearly visible. Toluidine blue, magnification: ×20

highlighted as a risk indicator for peri-implant mucositis [19]. Moreover, radiation therapy has been highlighted as a significant risk indicator for developing peri-implant mucositis [21]. With respect to peri-implant mucositis, the overall evidence should be considered weak for the following parameters: abutment surface characteristics, role of keratinized tissue, diabetes mellitus, genetics, gender and function time of implants. Some evidence was reported for the role of residual cement [19]. Moreover, systematic reviews indicate that subjects with a history of periodontitis are at greater risk for peri-implant disease [22].

From another review it was concluded that there is no obvious association between specific genetic polymorphism and dental implant failure in terms of biological complications, although a tendency should be underlined showing the potential link between IL-1 genotype and peri-implantitis [23]. Implants with a fixed prosthesis placed in the upper jaw along with bone augmentation procedures appeared to be more susceptible to peri-implant diseases [24]. Also bony defects following simultaneous augmentation of buccal dehiscences may increase the risk for peri-implantitis (LL DGZMK).

Finally, it has to be realized that peri-implantitis may be initiated and/or maintained by iatrogenic factors (e.g. inadequate restoration-abutments seating, overcountouring of restorations, implant malpositioning, technical complications). Moreover, bone loss induced at the time of implant placement by traumatizing the pristine bone beyond its adaptive capacity may also persist [17].

8.2.3 Clinical Findings

It was outlined that probing is essential for diagnosis of peri-implant diseases [18]. Therefore, the clinician must perform probing in order to monitor the peri-implant conditions and diagnose peri-implant disease. Probing using a conventional periodontal probe and using a light force (0.25 N) damages neither the mucosal attachment nor the implant [18]. Differences were seen in the pocket probing measurements at implants with or without the prosthetic reconstruction in place, and it was emphasized that the probing pocket depth following the removal of the prosthesis had a high correlation with the amount of bone loss at implants assessed during surgery [25]. Moreover, the profile of the implant might hinder probing at four surfaces per implant [18]. There are, in addition, implant (e.g. platform switching) and/or abutment designs at which probing may be difficult, and probing depth may underestimate the extent of the lesion [17].

Bleeding on probing indicates the presence of inflammation in the peri-implant mucosa and may be used as a predictor for loss of tissue support [18]. Bleeding may be associated with suppuration of pus, especially in deeper lesions [26]. Pus is a common finding in peri-implantitis sites [17]. An increase in probing depth over time is associated with the loss of attachment and supporting bone. The probing depth, the presence of bleeding on probing and suppuration should be assessed regularly for the diagnosis of peri-implant diseases [18]. Changes in the level of the crestal bone are seen in conjunction with bleeding on probing with or without concomitant deepening of peri-implant pockets. It is evident that recorded baseline data will be the reference from which the development of peri-implant disease can be recognized and followed in subsequent examinations [17]. However, the assessment of both bleeding on probing and probing depth scores at healthy implant sites is strongly influenced by the probing pressure and therefore bears a higher risk for false-positive outcomes when compared with natural teeth. If the probing pressure is not reported, it is impossible to estimate to what extent variations in probing forces may have contributed either to false-positive case definitions at baseline or false-negative outcomes after therapy [27].

From a clinical point of view, there are two different classes of peri-implant bone defects [28]. While Class I defects featured well-defined intrabony components, Class II defects were characterized by consistent horizontal bone loss (supraalveolar defects). In particular, human defects were most frequently circumferential (55.3%). In 80% of cases, Class I and Class II defects are combined [28].

A recent study identified that bacteria commonly associated with periodontitis were highly prevalent in peri-implantitis. Thus, specifically *T. forsythia* was found in 49% at implants with peri-implantitis and at 15% at implants with healthy conditions [29]. Therefore, microbiologic diagnosis is not regarded as prerequisite for therapy. Specific inflammatory cytokines in peri-implant crevicular fluid (PICF), such as IL-1β and TNF-α, can be used as additional criteria for a more robust diagnosis of healthy versus infected tissues. However, once the inflammatory process is installed, no differences were found between peri-implant mucositis and peri-implantitis [30]. Similarly, in a cross-sectional study, the potential of peri-implant crevicular fluid (PICF) analytes was evaluated to discriminate between peri-implant health and disease using a multi-biomarker approach [31]. Therefore, PICF samples from the mesiobuccal site of every implant (n = 145) from 52 subjects with peri-implantitis were collected, and the levels of 20 biomarkers were measured. Finally, there were statistically significant differences between healthy and diseased implants for 12/20 biomarkers. It was concluded that PICF biomarkers might help discriminate peri-implant health from disease. However, it was outlined that analysis of PICF is not a clinically useful diagnostic parameter for peri-implant disease [18].

8.2.4 Radiographic Findings

To establish baseline, a radiograph should be obtained to determine alveolar bone levels after physiologic remodelling, and peri-implant probing assessments performed [17]. Furthermore, when changes in the clinical parameters indicate disease (bleeding on probing, increased probing depth), the clinician is encouraged to take a radiograph to evaluate possible bone loss.

The bone level assessments are generally based on standardized periapical radiographs, taken with the use of an individualized radiograph holder [32]. Due to their two-dimensional nature, geometric distortions and anatomical superimpositions, the diagnostic value of intra-oral radiography is limited. Accordingly, the intraoperatively measured peri-implant bone levels were more apical than the radiographic bone levels [33, 34].

Peri-implant mucositis describes an inflammatory lesion that resides in the mucosa, while peri-implantitis also affects the supporting bone [18]. Early peri-implant bone resorption can be caused by remodelling that may be unrelated to infection and is not necessarily peri-implantitis. Long-term monitoring of implant performance should not be based on radiographs taken directly after implant placement but should rather relate to recordings obtained 3 months after completion of treatment, once tissue homeostasis has been established [6]. Assessing radiographs of implant patients, the intra-observer agreement was good or very good (weighted kappa statistic between 0.72 and 0.82), while the interobserver agreement was predominantly moderate (weighted kappa statistic between 0.58 and 0.62) [35].

Several authors have proposed other techniques to measure the bone level around implants, such as cone beam computed tomography (CBCT) or panoramic radiographs. CBCT allows the buccal and oral aspects of the implant to be viewed, but images may be altered by the presence of artefacts [36]. However, CBCT may represent an accurate diagnostic tool to estimate the histological extent of advanced peri-implantitis defects [37]. Panoramic radiographs show worse results than peri-apical radiographs because of their lower spatial resolution and nonlinear distortions [38].

8.3 Therapy of Peri-implant Mucositis

The goal in non-surgical therapy of peri-implant mucositis is to eliminate or significantly reduce the amounts of oral pathogens that allows healing and re-establishment of a clinically healthy condition.

8.3.1 Non-surgical Treatment of Peri-implant Mucositis

Literature has reported on the adjunctive effect of antimicrobial compounds (chlorhexidine, triclosan and essential oils) in the treatment of peri-implant mucositis. These studies have used short evaluation times (3–8 months) and share the problems of small sample sizes, the lack of a clear definition of the problem investigated (peri-implant mucositis) and incomplete registration of periodontal status in the studied samples [39]. Nevertheless, the endpoint of non-surgical therapy of mucositis should be the resolution of peri-implant mucosal inflammation (frequency distribution of resolved lesions) as determined by the absence of bleeding upon probing. As secondary outcomes, probing pocket depth reductions and outcomes assessing host–parasite interactions (presence of inflammatory biomarkers in peri-implant fluid and/or microbiological assessment of subgingival plaque samples) may be employed [39].

Despite clinically important improvements, a complete resolution of clinical signs indicating peri-implant mucositis may not be expected by any of the treatment and maintenance protocols investigated [27]. Test (i.e. alternative or adjunctive methods for biofilm removal, adjunctive antiseptic therapy or adjunctive antibiotic therapy) and control treatments were commonly associated with residual gingival index (GI) and/or bleeding scores at 3–12 months after therapy [16].

8.3.1.1 Alternative or Adjunctive Measures for Biofilm Removal

Schwarz reported on studies dealing with alternative or adjunctive measures for biofilm removal [16]. In particular, clinical efficacy of adjunctive air polishing (glycine powder) was compared to oral hygiene instructions and mechanical debridement using either ultrasonic scalers or hand instruments [32, 40]. Both test and control groups were associated with significant improvements in mean bleeding index and probing depth scores after therapy. When evaluating absolute values at 6 months, mean bleeding index and probing depth scores were significantly lower following adjunctive air polishing to Teflon curettes [32]. Riben Grundström et al.

compared a repeated (3 and 6 months) monotherapy using an air-abrasive device to ultrasonic scaling [41]. After a healing period of 12 months, both groups revealed comparable bleeding on probing reductions and frequencies of diseased sites.

8.3.1.2 Adjunctive Antiseptic/Antibiotic Therapy

Clinical efficacy of adjunctive antiseptic therapy to oral hygiene instructions and mechanical debridement was assessed. Strooker and coworkers assessed the adjunctive application of phosphoric acid gel to carbon curettes and rubber cup polishing, which was provided once every month in both groups. At 5 months, test sites revealed a significantly higher reduction in mean gingival index and colony-forming units when compared with control sites, respectively [42]. Porras and coworkers [43] compared oral hygiene instructions plus mechanical debridement with and without local pocket irrigation using chlorhexidine digluconate plus topical chlorhexidine digluconate gel application plus chlorhexidine digluconate mouthwash (twice for 10 days). At 3 months, mean mucosal bleeding, bleeding scores and microbiological parameters did not significantly differ between test and control groups. However, the test group revealed a significantly higher change in mean probing depth scores [43].

In another randomized clinical trial, topical chlorhexidine gel application plus full mouth disinfection plus chlorhexidine mouthrinse (2×/day) and tonsil spraying (1×/day) for 14 days was compared with oral hygiene instructions plus mechanical debridement (plastic scaler plus polyether ether ketone-coated ultrasonic instruments) plus full mouth scaling alone. While both treatment procedures were associated with significant probing depth reductions at 8 months, the bleeding on probing scores did not significantly differ to baseline in both groups [44].

The efficacy of non-surgical therapy for the management of peri-implant diseases at a two-piece zirconium implant system was assessed recently [45]. In this study, 17 patients (24 implants) were diagnosed with peri-implant mucositis and received mechanical debridement plus local antiseptic therapy using chlorhexidine digluconate (manual debridement plus chlorhexidine), while 17 patients (21 implants) diagnosed with peri-implantitis were assigned to Er:YAG laser therapy. Resolution of peri-implant mucositis and peri-implantitis was obtained in 9/17 (52.9%) ($p = 0.001$) and 5/17 (29.4%) ($p = 0.02$) of the patients, respectively. Due to these results, it was concluded that non-surgical treatment of either peri-implant mucositis using manual debridement plus chlorhexidine or peri-implantitis using Er:YAG laser therapy at zirconia implants was associated with significant short-term clinical improvements. A complete disease resolution, however, was not achieved in the majority of the patients.

Adjunctive efficacy of controlled topical tetracycline HCl application in the treatment of infection-associated peri-implant mucositis or mucosal hyperplasia was assessed in a clinical case series [46]. Control implants did not receive any other therapy aside from scaling. Scaling plus tetracycline HCl demonstrated a trend towards a reduction of bleeding on probing scores; scaling alone had no effect on bleeding on probing scores. In both groups, plaque index scores were slightly reduced at 4 weeks but returned to baseline values at 12 weeks. Another randomized clinical trial compared non-surgical treatment of peri-implant mucositis with or without systemic antibiotics [47]. Therefore, a total of 45 patients were randomly allocated to either oral hygiene instructions plus mechanical debridement (titanium curettes plus rubber polishing) plus systemic antibiotic medication (Azithromycin® 500 mg day 1 and 250 mg days 2–4) and were followed during 6 months. No short-term differences were found between study groups. It was concluded that clinical improvements observed at 6 months may be attributed to improvements in oral hygiene.

According to a meta-analysis by Schwarz and coworkers for non-surgical treatment of peri-implant mucositis—adjunctive antiseptics/antibiotics [16], the weighted mean difference between test and control treatments amounted in bleeding and probing scores to −8.16% and −0.15 mm, not favouring local antiseptic or antibiotic (i.e. local and systemic) therapy as an adjunct to mechanical debridement. Egger's linear regression method revealed symmetrical plots for changes in BOP and PD thus suggesting the absence of publication bias.

8.4 Therapy of Peri-implantitis

8.4.1 Non-surgical Treatment of Peri-implantitis

The goal in non-surgical therapy of peri-implantitis is to eliminate or significantly reduce the amounts of oral pathogens that allow healing and re-establishment of a clinically healthy condition [26]. Using conventional means of therapy, eradication of pathogens by mechanical means on implant surfaces with threads and often with rough surface structures is difficult [48]. Treatment models, such as scaling and root planing, effectively used to treat teeth with periodontitis, cannot be used in the same way on rough threaded implant surfaces. The implant rough surface structure also provides the bacteria with "protected areas" inaccessible to conventional mechanical removal [26].

In studies dealing with non-surgical treatment, peri-implantitis was commonly defined by bleeding on probing and radiographic bone loss. However, intervention studies have used different case definitions for peri-implantitis and have small sample sizes, along with short evaluation periods and a lack of a clear description of the periodontal status of the sample studied [39]. Moreover, reference points (i.e. baseline radiographs) and thresholds used to identify bone level changes were either not specified [49–51] or exhibited large variations [16, 26, 52–59]. A common finding in the reported studies was reductions in probing depths and bleeding on probing following the test and control interventions [39]. Radiographic bone level changes as treatment outcome were merely assessed in three studies [16, 26, 54, 56]. Despite significant improvements in all of the clinical and microbiological parameters investigated, test (i.e. alternative methods for biofilm removal, adjunctive antiseptic therapy or adjunctive antibiotic therapy) and control treatments were commonly associated with residual bleeding on probing scores at 3–12 months after therapy [16].

8.4.1.1 Alternative Measures for Biofilm Removal

For several years, an air-abrasive method for the removal of bacterial plaque on tooth surfaces has been in use [60]. This method has also been used in the treatment of peri-implantitis [61]. Air-polishing devices using an amino acid glycine have been proven to be effective in removing bacterial biofilm structures; therefore, a 25 μm hydrophobic powder and a flexible tip allowing access to implant pockets with less biokinetic pressure than the original device for supragingival polishing were shown to be of value [26]. Accordingly, no serious adverse events were identified in subjects treated with the air-abrasive device [26].

Several publications reported on the efficacy of alternative measures for biofilm removal. Among these, an ultrasonic device was used with a hydroxyapatite fluid polish [54, 55], whereas two studies reported on erbium-doped yttrium aluminium garnet (Er:YAG) laser monotherapy [51, 62] and another two publications on glycine powder air polishing [53, 58]. One study compared Er:YAG laser monotherapy versus air polishing [26]. At 3 months after therapy, non-surgical ultrasonic debridement was associated with a reduction in mean bleeding on probing scores, whereas these values further increased at control sites (i.e. carbon fibre curettes). However, these differences, as well as those noted for mean probing depth and radiographic bone level changes, did not reach statistical significance between groups [54]. Renvert and coworkers [55] also failed to identify any significance between group differences in mean bleeding index and probing depth reductions at 6 months when comparing ultrasonic scaling with mechanical debridement using titanium curettes. Furthermore, both procedures did not reduce bacterial load [48].

Moreover, efficacy of Er:YAG laser monotherapy was compared to that of mechanical debridement using carbon fibre curettes plus adjunctive local antiseptic chlorhexidine irrigation/application [51, 62]. After 6 months of healing, Er:YAG laser application was associated with significantly lower mean BOP scores than the control treatment. However, these improvements failed to reach statistical significance at 12 months, particularly at advanced sites [51, 62]. Glycine powder air polishing resulted in a significantly higher reduction of mean bleeding on probing scores at 3, 6 and 12 months when compared with mechanical debridement plus local antiseptic therapy using chlorhexidine [53, 58]. At more advanced sites, Er:YAG laser monotherapy and glycine powder air polishing resulted in comparable bleeding on probing and probing depth reductions and crestal bone level changes but failed to reduce bacterial load [63]. With respect to a two-piece zirconium implant system, it was reported that non-surgical treatment of peri-implantitis using Er:YAG laser at zirconia implants was associated with significant short-term clinical improvements. A complete disease resolution, however, was not achieved in the majority of the patients [45].

According to a meta-analysis by Schwarz and coworkers for non-surgical treatment of peri-implantitis—alternative methods for biofilm removal [16]—the weighted mean difference in bleeding on probing scores between test and control groups amounted to −23.12% favouring alternative methods (i.e. Er:YAG laser, glycine air polishing) for biofilm removal over mechanical debridement. Weighted mean difference in probing depth scores between test and control groups amounted to −0.49 mm not favouring alternative methods (i.e. Er:YAG laser, glycine air polishing, ultrasonic system) for biofilm removal over mechanical debridement. Moreover, Egger's linear regression method suggested the absence of any publication bias.

8.4.1.2 Adjunctive Antiseptic/Antibiotic Therapy

In a multicentre, randomized, double-blind, parallel, two-arm clinical trial, 60 patients (77 implants) were included with probing depth 6–10 mm and bone loss ≥2 mm around 1–2 implants to evaluate the efficacy of adjunctive antiseptic therapy to ultrasonic debridement. One to two weeks following surface debridement of the implant/s and the two adjacent teeth using ultrasonic instruments, patients were randomized to receive matrix chips (placebo) or chlorhexidine chips (PerioC). Measurements and chip placement were repeated at weeks 2, 4, 6, 8, 12 and 18 until probing depth was reduced to ≤5 mm. At 6 months, chlorhexidine chips resulted in a significantly higher probing depth reduction than the placebo chips [49].

Moreover, adjunctive local antibiotic therapy was compared to mechanical debridement. In particular, minocycline microspheres were either applied once at baseline [57] or repeatedly [56] at 30 and 90 days and compared with mechanical debridement and local antiseptic therapy using chlorhexidine gel (1.0%). As a result, repeated administration of a local antibiotic as an adjunct to the mechanical treatment of peri-implantitis lesions demonstrated improvements in probing depths that were significantly different from controls and were sustained for 6 months. However, radiographic and microbiological analyses failed to reveal any significant differences between both groups. Therefore, adjunctive use of minocycline microspheres was considered beneficial in the treatment of peri-implant lesions, but the treatment may have to be repeated.

In another study, for 2–18 weeks before week 0, all patients had been treated for peri-implantitis, including motivation, instruction in oral hygiene and implant scaling with a hand plastic instrument (Fig. 8.2). They were then randomly allocated to

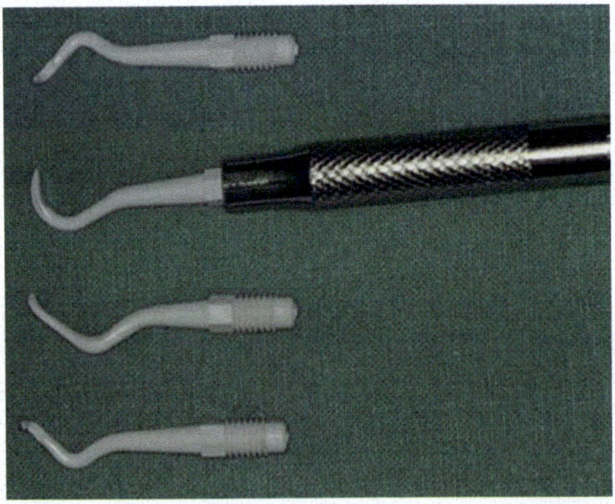

Fig. 8.2 Hand plastic instrument for implant scaling (Fa. Hu-Friedy, Chicago, USA)

continue with this treatment or to have in addition mechanical debridement and local application of doxycycline hyclate 10% (trade mark Atridox®) which slowly release doxycycline. Patients treated with doxycycline hyclate 10% showed a significantly greater gain in mean probing attachment levels (0.6 mm) than those not treated with doxycycline hyclate 10%. Only subjects treated with doxycycline hyclate 10% had a significant gain in mean bleeding on probing [52].

Finally, adjunctive local antibiotic therapy (minocycline microspheres) was compared to adjunctive antimicrobial photodynamic therapy. At 12 months, both test and control groups were associated with significant but comparable clinical, microbiological and immunological improvements [59, 64].

According to a meta-analysis by Schwarz and coworkers for non-surgical treatment of peri-implantitis—adjunctive antiseptic/antibiotic therapy [16]—the weighted mean difference in bleeding scores between test and control groups amounted to −16.53% favouring local antibiotic therapy as an adjunct to mechanical debridement. Weighted mean difference in probing depth scores between test and control groups amounted to −0.829 mm not favouring antiseptic/antibiotic therapy as an adjunct to mechanical debridement. Egger's linear regression method suggested the absence of any publication bias.

With respect to non-surgical treatment of peri-implantitis, literature demonstrated a limited efficacy at "deep sites." In particular, several studies reported on increasing bleeding on probing scores between 3 and 12 months following non-surgical treatment of "severe" peri-implantitis sites using either mechanical debridement, adjunctive aPDT (Fig. 8.3a–e), Er:YAG laser monotherapy or glycine powder air polishing. The efficacy of all treatment procedures investigated was higher at "moderately" deep sites [16, 53, 58, 62, 65].

8.4.2 Surgical Treatment of Peri-implantitis

According to Mombelli and coworkers [66], surgical intervention in deep peri-implant lesions with extensive bacterial surface contamination may provide better access and may allow further therapies to change the peri-implant tissue morphology, to stabilize the site during the healing phase or to promote the regeneration of bone. Clinical efficacy and safety of treatment procedures has been shown in the beagle dog model (Fig. 8.4a–e) [67].

There are several studies in which the efficacy of surgical therapies for the treatment of peri-implantitis was assessed. However, most intervention studies have used different case definitions for peri-implantitis and have, in common, small sample sizes and the lack of a clear description of the periodontal and smoking status of studied sample [39], and defect configurations (i.e. supra-/intrabony defects) [28] were rarely reported.

At present [16], for surgical treatment of peri-implantitis, open debridement is recommended, employing either alternative measures for surface decontamination [61, 68–70], adjunctive resective [71] or augmentative therapy [50, 61, 72–83].

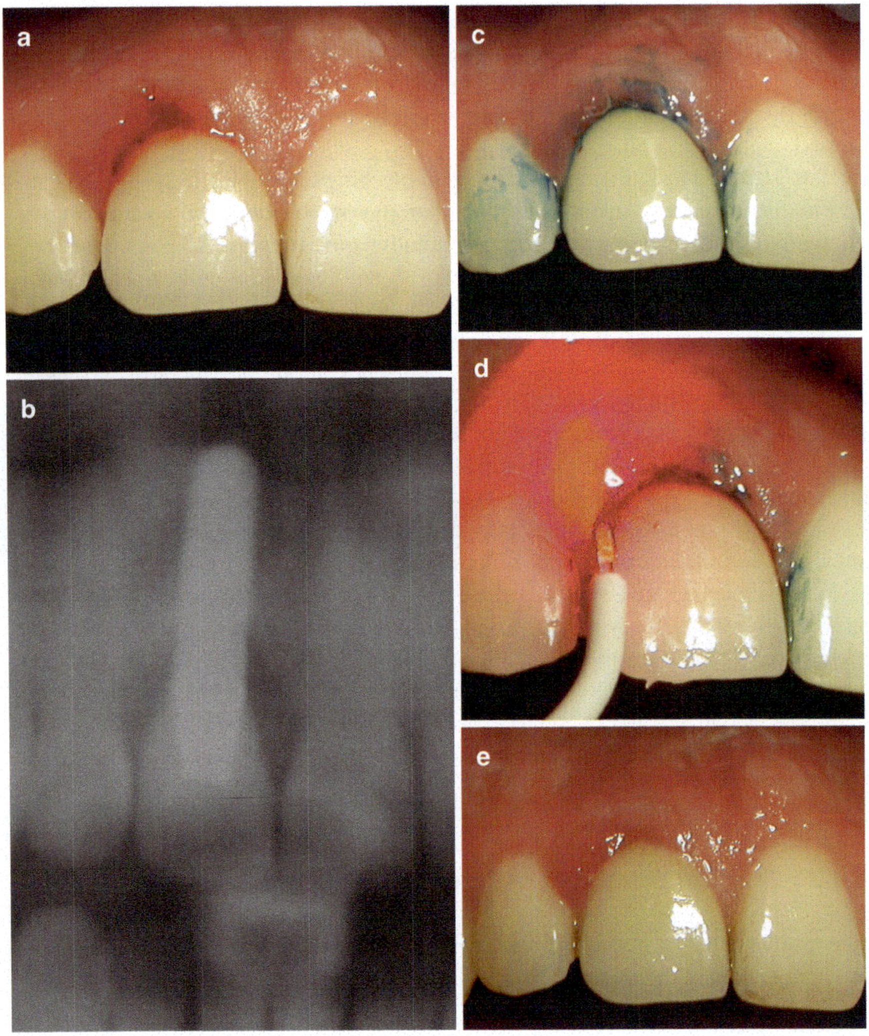

Fig. 8.3 (**a**) Clinical aspect of a chronic peri-implantitis lesion. (**b**) Radiograph showing vertical bony defects indicating progressive peri-implant bone resorption. (**c**) Clinical aspect following application of a photosensitizer. (**d**) Non-surgical intervention: application of diode laser light. (**e**) Clinical aspect 6 months after therapy. Local infection visible

8.4.2.1 Alternative Measures for Surface Decontamination

Deppe and coworkers [61] assessed the clinical efficacy of carbon dioxide laser decontamination used as an adjunct to resective flap surgery plus air polishing (control) (Fig. 8.5). While the test treatment improved the clinical outcomes over the control measure at 4 months, mean sulcus bleeding index and probing depth values were comparable in both groups at about 5 years.

Similarly, neither a 980-nm diode laser [70] nor 2% chlorhexidine solution [68] nor 0.12% chlorhexidine plus 0.05% cetylpyridinium chloride [69], used as adjuncts to mechanical open flap debridement, resulted in statistically significant better clinical or radiographic results as compared to controls (access flaps plus plastic curettes plus sterilized gauzes soaked in saline [70], 0.12% chlorhexidine plus 0.05% cetylpyridinium chloride [68] or placebo solution [69]).

According to a meta-analysis by Schwarz and coworkers for non-surgical treatment of peri-implantitis—alternative measures for surface decontamination [16, 68, 69], the weighted mean difference in bleeding on probing and probing depth scores between test and control groups amounted to 5.61% and 0.22 mm, not favouring alternative (i.e. 0.12% chlorhexidine plus 0.05% cetylpyridinium chloride) over conventional (i.e. 2.0% chlorhexidine) measures for surface decontamination.

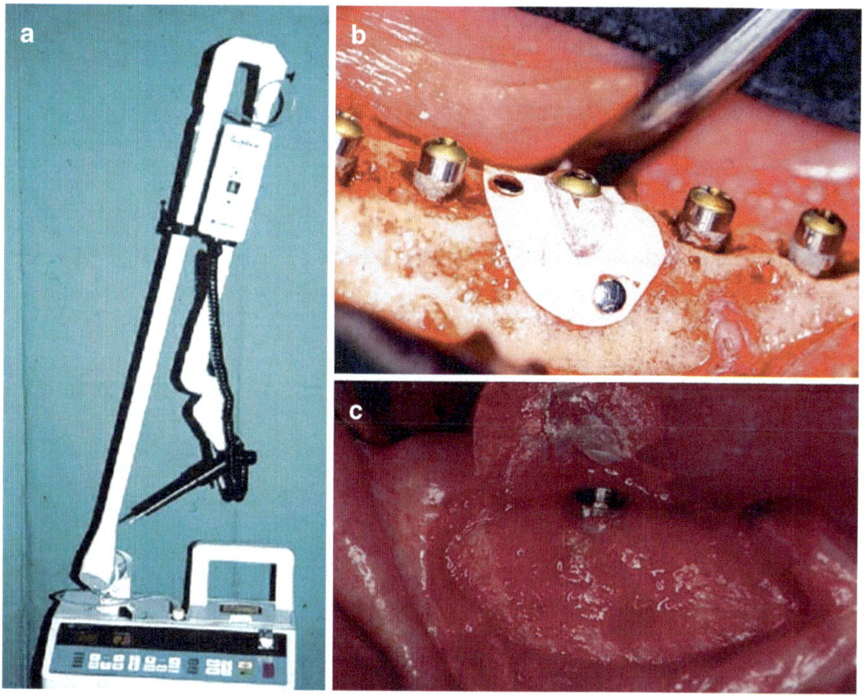

Fig. 8.4 (**a**) Medical CO_2 laser ($\lambda = 10.6$ µm) (Sharplan, D-Freising). (**b**) Experimentally induced peri-implant defects following CO_2 laser decontamination, with or without application of a non-resorbable membrane. (**c**) Clinical aspect at re-entry. Complete closure of the defect. (**d**) Section of an implant after CO_2 laser-assisted therapy without membrane: large areas of newly formed bone in direct implant contact (new bone stained darker than old bone). Toluidine blue, magnification ×5. Length of bar: 50 µm. (**e**) Section of an implant after CO_2 laser-assisted therapy, concomitantly treated with a non-resorbable membrane. Reappositioned bone ending at the roughened surface. Toluidine blue, magnification ×5

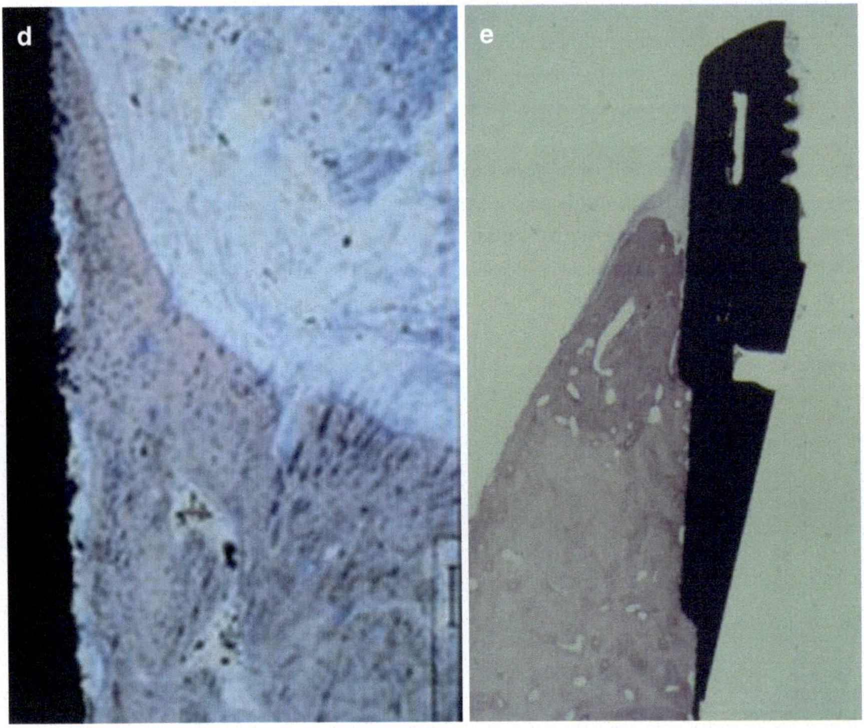

Fig. 8.4 (continued)

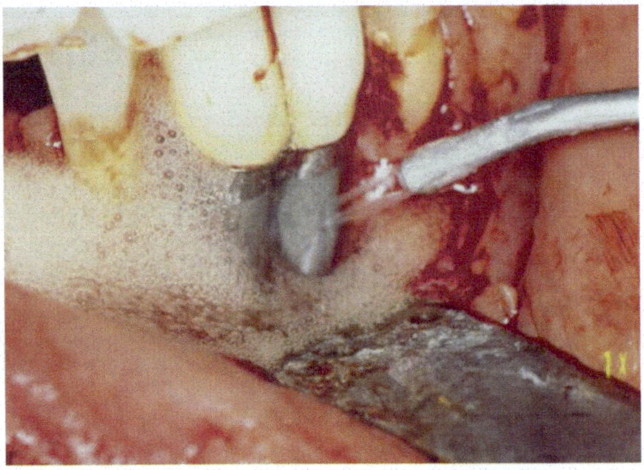

Fig. 8.5 Decontamination of implant surfaces with an airflow device

8.4.2.2 Adjunctive Resective Therapy

Clinical efficacy of implantoplasty (diamond/Arkansas burs plus silicone polishers) was assessed when used as an adjunct to open flap debridement plus bone recontouring plus apical flap repositioning [71]. This resective therapy resulted in significantly higher mean mucosal recessions (1.64 ± 1.29 vs. 2.3 ± 1.45 mm) but no

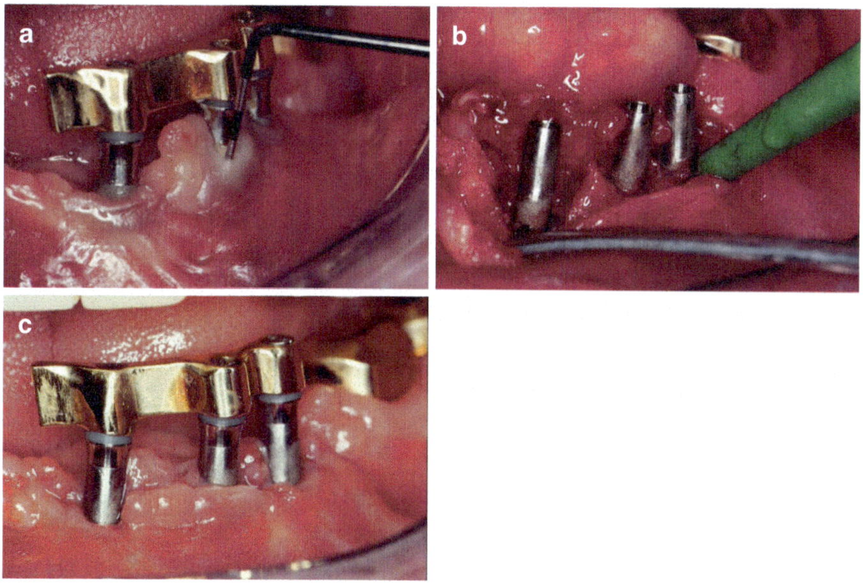

Fig. 8.6 (**a**) Chronically progressive peri-implant bone loss with severe probing depth. (**b**) Clinical aspect following implantoplasty and after CO_2 laser decontamination. (**c**) Clinical result 4 months after therapy. No clinical signs of infection

pseudopocket formation [71]. While test sites were associated with stable radiographic bone levels at 3 years, the interproximal bone loss at control sites amounted to 1.45–1.54 mm [84]. Therefore, at 24 months, all patients from the control group had to be discontinued from the study due to persistent active signs of peri-implant inflammation which was associated with elevated bleeding index and probing depth scores when compared with the test group [16].

According to a meta-analysis by Schwarz and coworkers for surgical treatment of peri-implantitis (i.e. open flap with and without soft tissue resection), the weighted mean in bleeding on probing [68, 69, 82] and probing depth [61, 68, 69, 82] reductions amounted to 34.81% and 1.75 mm [16] (Fig. 8.6a–c).

8.4.2.3 Adjunctive Augmentative Therapy

Limited evidence exists on the efficacy of regenerative treatment of peri-implantitis [72]. For the purpose of adjunctive augmentative therapy, bone fillers (i.e. alloplastic, xenogenic, autogenous) have been proposed. Interestingly, it was stated that porous titanium granules (PTG) may have potential as an osteoconductive bone graft substitute to treat peri-implant osseous defects. In a prospective, randomized, case-control, clinical 12-month study, open flap debridement and surface decontamination with titanium curettes and 24% ethylenediaminetetraacetic acid gel ($n = 16$) were compared to the same protocol but with the addition of PTG ($n = 16$) [82]. One-, two- and three-wall intrabony defects were included. Patients were given amoxicillin and metronidazole 3 days before surgery and for 7 days afterwards. Implants were submerged and allowed to heal for 6 months. However, 12/16 control and 13/16 test sites revealed a premature exposure during the submerged healing phase of 6 months. Accordingly, both treatment modalities demonstrated significant improvements in probing pocket depth, but significant differences between groups were not observed. Nevertheless, reconstruction with PTG resulted in significantly better radiographic peri-implant defect fill compared with controls and showed an increase in implant stability quotient (ISQ) of 1.6 units, compared with a decrease of 0.7 ISQ for the control group [82]. In addition, matrix metalloproteinase-8 levels were measured using the Quantikine Human Total MMP-8 (DMP800) ELISA. Again, no differences in clinical parameter or bone marker levels between test and control groups were found [85].

Different augmentation protocols and various methods for surface decontamination, several bone fillers (i.e. alloplastic, xenogenic, autogenous) (Fig. 8.7a–f) and barrier membranes (synthetic, native collagen) (Fig. 8.8a–e) were compared over a period of up to 5 years [50, 61, 72–83]. In two case series, the 2-year results and the 4-year clinical outcomes obtained following treatment of peri-implantitis

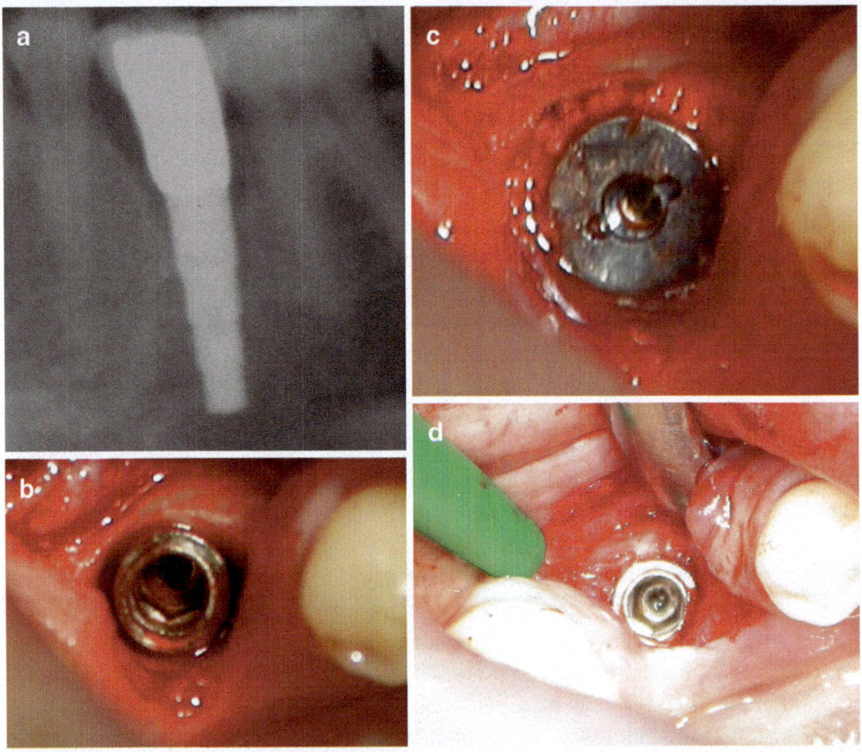

Fig. 8.7 (**a**) Chronically progressive peri-implant bone loss with severe probing depth. (**b**) Clinical aspect following CO_2 laser decontamination. (**c**) Augmentation of the defect with resorbable β-TCP (Cerasorb®, Riemser AG, D-Greifswald). (**d**) Re-entry 4 months after therapy. Complete closure of the defect. (**e**) Radiographic result 5 years after therapy. (**f**) Clinical result 5 years after therapy

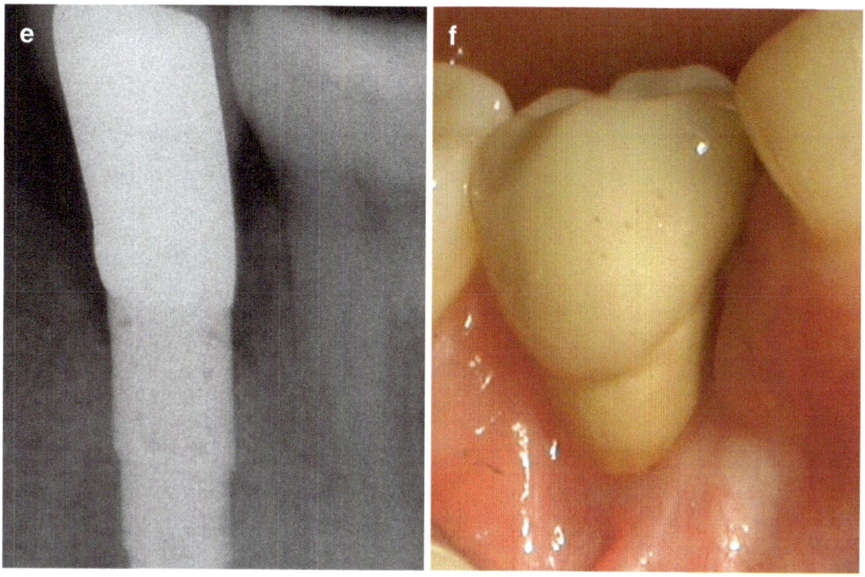

Fig. 8.7 (continued)

lesions using either a nanocrystalline hydroxyapatite or a natural bone mineral in combination with a collagen membrane were evaluated. Both treatment procedures have shown efficacy over a period of 24 months [77, 83]; however, the application of bone fillers with a collagen membrane may result in an improved outcome of healing [81]. These results were superior to autogenous bone or bovine-derived xenograft (both with placement of a collagen membrane) [72]. In the latter study, bovine xenograft provided more radiographic bone fill than autogenous bone. However, success for both surgical regenerative procedures was limited. Nevertheless, decreases in bleeding on probing and probing depth scores and suppuration were observed.

Several studies indicated that neither barrier membranes nor the method of surface decontamination may improve clinical outcomes following surgical debridement [61, 75, 83, 86]. It was emphasized that differences between the three surgical treatment protocols (flap surgery plus autogenous bone grafts alone (controls) plus non-resorbable (test 1) or bioabsorbable barriers (test 2) and supportive antimicrobial therapy) did not affect the treatment outcomes after 3 years [86]. In contrast, it was pointed out that defect configuration may have an impact on the clinical outcome following surgical regenerative therapy of peri-implantitis lesions. While Class Ie defects seem to be promising in conjunction with natural bone mineral in combination with a collagen membrane, Class Ib and Class Ic may be considered as unfavourable [79]. Furthermore, surface characteristics (TPS, Control or SLA, test) may have an impact on the clinical outcome. Following surgical debridement, disinfection of the contaminated surfaces and grafting with a bovine-derived xenograft, the flap was sutured around the non-submerged implant. One-year follow-up

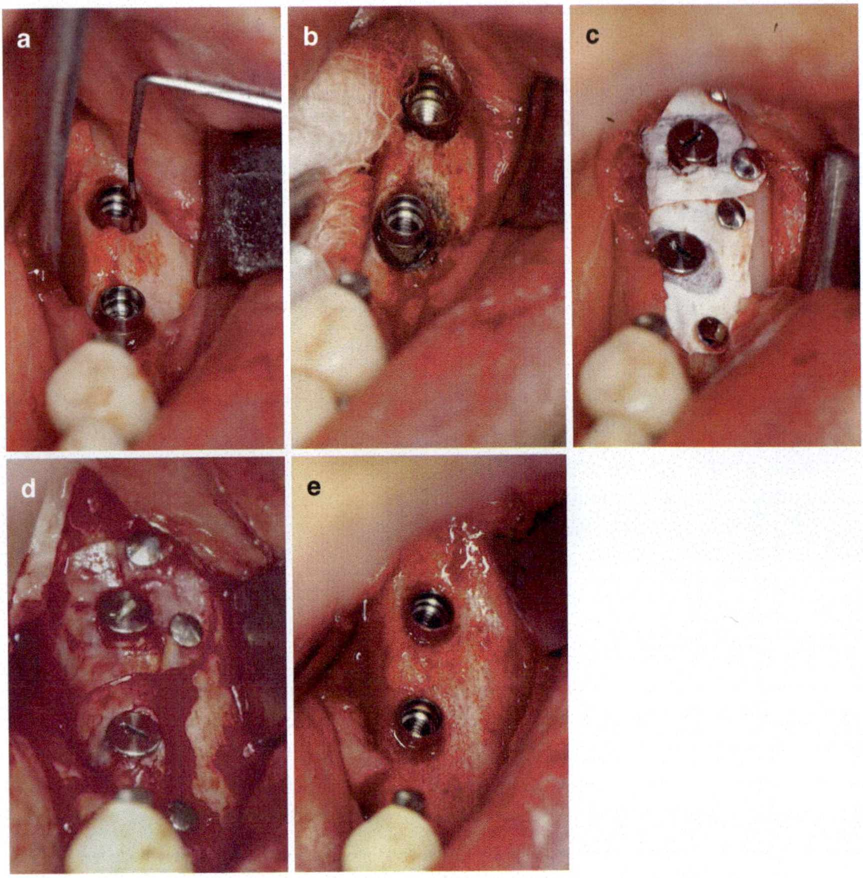

Fig. 8.8 (**a**) Chronically progressive peri-implant bone loss with severe probing depth. (**b**) Clinical aspect following CO_2 laser decontamination. (**c**) Augmentation of the defect with non-resorbable ePTFE membrane (Gore-Tex®, WL Gore & Associates GmbH, D-Putzbrunn). (**d**) Re-entry 4 months after therapy. Membranes without clinical signs of infection. (**e**) Clinical result following removal of membranes. Complete closure of the defects

demonstrated clinical and radiographic improvements. Probing depths were significantly reduced by 2.1 ± 1.2 mm in the control implants and by 3.4 ± 1.7 mm in the test implants [73].

According to a meta-analysis by Schwarz and coworkers for surgical treatment of peri-implantitis—adjunctive augmentative therapy [16]—the weighted mean in bleeding on probing [72, 77, 79, 80, 82] and probing depth [50, 61, 72–83] reductions following adjunctive augmentative therapy amounted to 50.73% and 2.20 mm, respectively. In detail, outcomes of therapy were mainly influenced by the type of bone filler (i.e. a slowly resorbing bovine-derived mineral was superior to autogenous bone and an alloplastic material), defect characteristics (i.e. circumferential-type defects were superior to dehiscence-type defects) and implant surface characteristics (i.e. moderately rough surfaces were superior to rough surfaces) [16].

A randomized, controlled clinical trial was primarily designed to investigate the impact of surface decontamination on the outcome of a combined surgical resective/regenerative therapy of moderate to advanced peri-implantitis defects [78]. Therefore, mucoperiosteal flaps were raised buccally and orally by means of intracrevicular incisions under local anaesthesia. Subsequently, all granulation tissue was completely removed from the defect area and the implant surfaces by means of plastic curettes. Implantoplasty at both buccally (i.e. Classes Ib and Ic) and supracrestally (i.e. Class II) exposed implant surfaces was performed in a way as to completely planish the threatened areas and smoothen the structured implant surface using diamant burs and Arkansas stones under copious irrigation with sterile saline. Decontamination was performed randomly with an Er:YAG laser device or plastic curettes plus cotton pellets plus sterile saline. In both groups, the intrabony component was augmented with a natural bone mineral and covered with a collagen membrane. After 6 months, the study failed to demonstrate a significant impact of the method of surface decontamination on the clinical outcome following combined surgical therapy of advanced peri-implantitis lesions [78]. The 2-year [83], and 4-year [77] clinical outcomes obtained following combined surgical resective/regenerative therapy of advanced peri-implantitis were not influenced by the method of surface decontamination.

In conclusion, most studies documented reductions in bleeding on probing and probing depth scores as well radiographic defect fill. However, complete fill of the bony defect seems not to be a predictable result [73].

With respect to mucosal recessions following surgical therapy of peri-implantitis, there are very limited data evaluating different treatment options for covering peri-implant soft tissue recessions, and thus, the long-term stability outcomes following these procedures are still unknown [87]. Accordingly, the limited available data indicate that only shallow peri-implant mucosal recessions (e.g. up to 2 mm) may be treated successfully by means of a coronally advanced flap and subepithelial connective tissue graft or with guided bone regeneration, while no data are available supporting the possibility of covering deep and large peri-implant mucosal recessions.

8.5 Apical Peri-implantitis

A specific form of peri-implantitis is the apical or retrograde peri-implantitis (RPI). Dental implants may not osseointegrate in sites of endodontic failure. This may occur as a result colonization by various anaerobic and facultative bacterial species [88]. Although RPI is not a common sequela of dental implant surgery, its prevalence has been reported in the literature to be 0.26% [89]. If an implant is placed in a site where vegetative bacteria are residing, the implant may fail to integrate if a bacterial colonization proceeds coronally. Especially, *Enterococcus faecalis* may be the most important germ in these types of implant failures. When teeth adjacent to the implant site have a previous history of root canal therapy, incidence of RPI is reported to increase to 7.8% [89]. Accordingly, a distance of at least 2 mm space between implant and adjacent tooth is needed to decrease incidence of apical RPI, with minimum 4 weeks between completion of endodontic treatment and actual implant placement [89]. Data from a review demonstrate that RPI was diagnosed between 1 week and 4 years after implant placement [89].

Both immediate implant placement and waiting for postextraction healing may allow for the formation of bacterial vegetative forms or biofilms [88]. The implant surface may be colonized when the surface is exposed to the bacteria. According to a systematic review, the average time of the diagnosis of the pathology was found to be 26.07 weeks after implant placement [90]. With respect to therapy, regenerative treatment (45.2% of the cases) or implant removal (35.7% of the cases) was the most common treatment techniques used [90].

Further studies are needed to focus on histologic data around periapical microbiota to establish specific aetiology and differential diagnoses compared with marginal peri-implantitis and other implant-related conditions.

8.6 Clinical Implications

According to the German Society for Dental and Oral Medicine (DGZMK) [15], the following recommendations can be given at present [16]:

8.6.1 Non-surgical Treatment of Peri-implant Mucositis

Professional supportive care should be performed [1]. Professionally and patient-administered mechanical plaque control alone should be considered the standard of care in the management of peri-implant mucositis. Therapy of peri-implant mucositis is a prerequisite for the prevention of peri-implantitis [91]. Alternative or adjunctive therapy may not improve the efficacy of professionally administered biofilm removal in reducing bleeding on probing, gingival index and probing depth scores at mucositis sites [27].

Despite clinically important improvements, a complete disease resolution may not be expected by any of the treatment protocols investigated [27]. Professional supportive care should be established according to the individual needs of the patient (e.g. 3-, 6- or 12-month recall intervals), and their compliance has to be confirmed [1].

When implant treatment is considered, patients should be informed on the risks for biological complications (peri-implant diseases) and the need for preventive care [1]. An individual risk assessment including systemic and local risk indicators should be performed, and modifiable risk factors, such as residual increased probing pocket depth in the remaining dentition or smoking, should be eliminated [1]. The correct fit of implant components and the suprastructure has to be ensured to avoid additional niches for biofilm adherence. If cemented implant restorations have been selected, the restoration margins should be located at the mucosal margin to allow meticulous removal of excess cement.

8.6.2 Non-surgical Treatment of Peri-implantitis

Alternative/adjunctive measures may improve the efficacy over/of conventional treatments (oral hygiene instructions plus mechanical debridement) at peri-implantitis sites [16]. Literature has shown evidence for alternative monotherapy with glycine powder air polishing, Er:YAG laser and adjunctive application of doxycycline, chlorhexidine chips and antimicrobial photodynamic therapy [16].

Clinical results of non-surgical treatment of peri-implantitis and maintenance of results for more than 6 months were limited, especially in cases with severe peri-implantitis (probing depth initially >7 mm) [26, 62, 65]. If the aim of the therapy cannot be yielded by non-surgical treatment of peri-implantitis, early surgical intervention, especially in severe peri-implant lesions, should be intended. Before therapy, an individual risk assessment including systemic and local risk indicators should be performed. The correct fit of implant components and the suprastructure has to be ensured to avoid additional niches for biofilm adherence.

8.6.3 Surgical Treatment of Peri-implantitis

The currently available evidence does not allow any firm specific recommendation for the surgical therapy of peri-implantitis [16]. During surgery, it is recommended to remove granulation tissue completely. Decontamination of the implant surface should be performed meticulously. However, there is no evidence for favouring alternative (i.e. chlorhexidine plus cetylpyridinium chloride) over conventional (i.e. chlorhexidine) measures for surface decontamination [16].

At present, there is no evidence for peri- and/or postoperative antibiotic medication. However, before the surgical intervention, a single-shot antibiotic prophylaxis may be of value. Augmentative measures following decontamination may result in radiographically visible filling of intraosseous defects [16]. The clinician must be aware that any surgical intervention may cause mucosal recessions postoperatively. For stabilization of peri-implant mucosa, soft tissue augmentation may be performed [92]. Mobile implants, irreversible technical complications, complex implant design such as hollow cylinders, recurrence of infection or infection of neighbouring tissues need explanation.

References

1. Jepsen S, Berglundh T, Genco R, Aass AM, Demirel K, Derks J, Figuero E, Giovannoli JL, Goldstein M, Lambert F, Ortiz-Vigon A, Polyzois I, Salvi GE, Schwarz F, Serino G, Tomasi C, Zitzmann NU. Primary prevention of peri-implantitis: managing periimplant mucositis. J Clin Periodontol. 2015;42(Suppl 16):S152–7.
2. Schmidt KE, Auschill TM, Heumann C, Frankenberger R, Eick S, Sculean A, Arweiler NB. Influence of different instrumentation modalities on the surface characteristics and biofilm formation on dental implant neck, in vitro. Clin Oral Implants Res. 2016;24:483–90.
3. Schwarz F, Sculean A, Engebretson SP, Becker J, Sager M. Animal models for peri-implant mucositis and peri-implantitis. Periodontol 2000. 2015e;68:168–81.
4. Derks J, Tomasi C. Peri-implant health and disease: a systematic review of current epidemiology. J Clin Periodontol. 2015;42(Suppl 16):S158–71.
5. Figuero E, Graziani F, Sanz I, Herrera D, Sanz M. Management of peri-implant mucositis and peri-implantitis. Periodontol 2000. 2014;66:255–73.
6. Klinge B, Meyle J, Working Group 2. Peri-implant tissue destruction. The Third EAO Consensus Conference 2012. Clin Oral Implants Res. 2012;23(Suppl 6):108–10.
7. Mombelli A, Müller N, Cionca N. The epidemiology of peri-implantitis. Clin Oral Implants Res. 2012a;23(Suppl 6):67–76.
8. Tomasi C, Derks J. Clinical research of peri-implant diseases: quality of reporting, case definitions and methods to study incidence, prevalence and risk factors of peri-implant diseases. J Clin Periodontol. 2012;39(Suppl 12):207–23.
9. Merli M, Bernardelli F, Giulianelli E, Toselli I, Moscatelli M, Pagliaro U, Nieri M. Inter-rater agreement in the diagnosis of mucositis and peri-implantitis. J Clin Periodontol. 2014;41:927–33.
10. Carcuac O, Berglundh T. Composition of human peri-implantitis and periodontitis lesions. J Dent Res. 2014;93:1083–8.
11. Salvi GE, Aglietta M, Eick S, Sculean A, Lang NP, Ramseier CA. Reversibility of experimental peri-implant mucositis compared with experimental gingivitis in humans. Clin Oral Implants Res. 2012;23:182–90.
12. Costa FO, Takenaka-Martinez S, Cota LO, Ferreira SD, Silva GL, Costa JE. Periimplant disease in subjects with and without preventive maintenance: a 5-year follow-up. J Clin Periodontol. 2012;39:173–81.
13. Zitzmann NU, Berglundh T, Ericsson I, Lindhe J. Spontaneous progression of experimentally induced periimplantitis. J Clin Periodontol. 2004;31:845–9.
14. Derks J, Schaller D, Håkansson J, jl W, Tomasi C, Berglundh T. Effectiveness of implant therapy analyzed in a Swedish population: prevalence of peri-implantitis. J Dent Res. 2016;95:43–9.
15. Schwarz F (2016) Die Behandlung periimplantärer Infektionen an Zahnimplantaten. S3-Leitlinie. AWMF-Registernummer: 083-023
16. Schwarz F, Schmucker A, Becker J. Efficacy of alternative or adjunctive measures to conventional treatment of peri-implant mucositis and peri-implantitis: a systematic review and meta-analysis. International Journal of Implant Dentistry. 2015a;1:22–56.
17. Lang NP, Berglundh T, Behalf of Working Group 4 of the Seventh European Workshop on Periodontology. Periimplant diseases: where are we now? – consensus of the seventh European workshop on periodontology. J Clin Periodontol. 2011b;38(Suppl. 11):178–81.
18. Lindhe J, Meyle J, Group D of European Workshop on Periodontology. Peri-implant diseases: consensus report of the sixth European workshop on periodontology. J Clin Periodontol. 2008;35(8 Suppl):282–5.
19. Renvert S, Polyzois I. Risk indicators for peri-implant mucositis: a systematic literature review. J Clin Periodontol. 2015;42(Suppl. 16):S172–86.

20. Lang NP, Bosshardt DD, Lulic M. Do mucositis lesions around implants differ from gingivitis lesions around teeth? J Clin Periodontol. 2011a;38(Suppl 11):182–7.
21. Karbach J, Callaway A, Kwon YD, d'Hoedt B, Al-Nawas B. Comparison of five parameters as risk factors for perimucositis. Int J Oral Maxillofac Implants. 2009;24:491–6.
22. Heitz-Mayfield LJ. Peri-implant diseases: diagnosis and risk indicators. J Clin Periodontol. 2008;35:292–304.
23. Dereka X, Mardas N, Chin S, Petrie A, Donos N. A systematic review on the association between genetic predisposition and dental implant biological complications. Clin Oral Implants Res. 2012;23:775–88.
24. Schwarz F, Becker K, Sahm N, Horstkemper T, Rousi K, Becker J. The prevalence of peri-implant diseases for two-piece implants with an internal tube-in-tube connection: a cross-sectional analysis of 512 implants. Clin Oral Implants Res. 2015d;28(1):24–8.
25. Serino G, Turri A, Lang NP. Probing at implants with peri-implantitis and its relation to clinical peri-implant bone loss. Clin Oral Implants Res. 2013;24:91–5.
26. Renvert S, Lindahl C, Roos Jansaker A-M, Persson GR. Treatment of peri-implantitis using Er:YAG laser or an air-abrasive device: a randomized clinical trial. J Clin Periodontol. 2011;38:65–73.
27. Schwarz F, Becker K, Sager M. Efficacy of professionally administered plaque removal with or without adjunctive measures for the treatment of peri-implant mucositis. A systematic review and meta-analysis. J Clin Periodontol. 2015b;42 Suppl 16:S202–13.
28. Schwarz F, Herten M, Sager M, Bieling K, Sculean A, Becker J. Comparison of naturally occurring and ligature-induced peri-implantitis bone defects in humans and dogs. Clin Oral Implants Res. 2007;18:161–70.
29. Persson GR, Renvert S. Cluster of bacteria associated with peri-implantitis. Clin Implant Dent Relat Res. 2014;16:783–93.
30. Faot F, Nascimento GG, Bielemann AM, Campao TD, Leite FR, Quirynen M. Can peri-implant crevicular fluid assist in the diagnosis of peri-implantitis? A systematic review and meta-analysis. J Periodontol. 2015;86:631–45.
31. Zani SR, Moss K, Shibli JA, Teixeira ER, de Oliveira Mairink R, Onuma T, Feres M, Teles RP. Peri-implant crevicular fluid biomarkers as discriminants of peri-implant health and disease. J Clin Periodontol. 2016;43:825–32.
32. De Siena F, Corbella S, Taschieri S, Del Fabbro M, Francetti L. Adjunctive glycine powder air-polishing for the treatment of peri-implant mucositis: an observational clinical trial. Int J Dent Hyg. 2015;13:170–6.
33. Deppe H, Wagenpfeil S, Donath K. Comparative value of attachment measurements in implant dentistry. Int J Oral Maxillofac Implants. 2004;19:208–15.
34. Garcıa-Garcıa M, Mir-Mari J, Benic GI, Figueiredo R, Valmaseda-Castellon E. Accuracy of periapical radiography in assessing bone level in implants affected by peri-implantitis: a cross-sectional study. J Clin Periodontol. 2016;43:85–91.
35. Kullman L, Al-Asfour A, Zetterqvist L, Andersson L. Comparison of radiographic bone height assessments in panoramic and intraoral radiographs of implant patients. Int J Oral Maxillofac Implants. 2007;22:96–100.
36. Schulze RK, Berndt D, d'Hoedt B. On cone-beam computed tomography artifacts induced by titanium implants. Clin Oral Implants Res. 2010;21:100–7.
37. Golubovic V, Mihatovic I, Becker J, Schwarz F. Accuracy of cone-beam computed tomography to assess the configuration and extent of ligature-induced peri-implantitis defects. A pilot study. Oral Maxillofac Surg. 2012;16:349–54.
38. Lam EWN, Ruprecht A, Yang J. Comparison of two-dimensional orthoradially reformatted computed tomography and panoramic radiography for dental implant treatment planning. J Prosthet Dent. 1995;74:42–6.
39. Sanz M, Chapple IL, Working Group 4 of the, V. E. W. o. P. Clinical research on periimplant diseases: consensus report of Working Group 4. J Clin Periodontol. 2012;39(Suppl 12):202–6.

40. Ji YJ, Tang ZH, Wang R, Cao J, Cao CF, Jin LJ. Effect of glycine powder air-polishing as an adjunct in the treatment of peri-implant mucositis: a pilot clinical trial. Clin Oral Implants Res. 2014;25:683–9.
41. Riben Grundström C, Norderyd O, Andre U, Renvert S. Treatment of peri-implant mucositis using a glycine powder air-polishing or ultrasonic device. A randomized clinical trial. J Clin Periodontol. 2015;42:462–9.
42. Strooker H, Rohn S, Van Winkelhoff AJ. Clinical and microbiologic effects of chemical versus mechanical cleansing in professional supportive implant therapy. Int J Oral Maxillofac Implants. 1998;13:845–50.
43. Porras R, Anderson GB, Caffesse R, Narendran S, Trejo PM. Clinical response to 2 different therapeutic regimens to treat peri-implant mucositis. J Periodontol. 2002;73:1118–25.
44. Thone-Mühling M, Swierkot K, Nonnenmacher C, Mutters R, Flores-de-Jacoby L, Mengel R. Comparison of two full-mouth approaches in the treatment of peri-implant mucositis: a pilot study. Clin Oral Implants Res. 2010;21:504–12.
45. Schwarz F, John G, Hegewald A, Becker J. Non-surgical treatment of peri-implant mucositis and peri-implantitis at zirconia implants: a prospective case series. J Clin Periodontol. 2015c;42:783–8.
46. Schenk G, Flemmig TF, Betz T, Reuther J, Klaiber B. Controlled local delivery of tetracycline HCl in the treatment of periimplant mucosal hyperplasia and mucositis. A controlled case series. Clin Oral Implants Res. 1997;8:427–33.
47. Hallstrom H, Persson GR, Lindgren S, Olofsson M, Renvert S. Systemic antibiotics and debridement of peri-implant mucositis. A randomized clinical trial. J Clin Periodontol. 2012;39:574–81.
48. Persson GR, Samuelsson E, Lindahl C, Renvert S. Mechanical non-surgical treatment of peri-implantitis: a single-blinded randomized longitudinal clinical study. II. Microbiological results. J Clin Periodontol. 2010;37:563–73.
49. Machtei EE, Frankenthal S, Levi G, Elimelech R, Shoshani E, Rosenfeld O, et al. Treatment of peri-implantitis using multiple applications of chlorhexidine chips: a double-blind, randomized multi-centre clinical trial. J Clin Periodontol. 2012;3:1198–205.
50. Schwarz F, Bieling K, Latz T, Nuesry E, Becker J. Healing of intrabony peri-implantitis defects following application of a nanocrystalline hydroxyapatite (Ostim) or a bovine-derived xenograft (Bio-Oss) in combination with a collagen membrane (Bio-Gide). A case series. J Clin Periodontol. 2006a;33:491–9.
51. Schwarz F, Sculean A, Rothamel D, Schwenzer K, Georg T, Becker J. Clinical evaluation of an Er:YAG laser for nonsurgical treatment of peri-implantitis: a pilot study. Clin Oral Implants Res. 2005;16:44–52.
52. Büchter A, Meyer U, Kruse-Losler B, Joos U, Kleinheinz J. Sustained release of doxycycline for the treatment of peri-implantitis: randomised controlled trial. Br J Oral Maxillofac Surg. 2004;42:439–44.
53. John G, Sahm N, Becker J, Schwarz F. Nonsurgical treatment of peri-implantitis using an air-abrasive device or mechanical debridement and local application of chlorhexidine. Twelve-month follow-up of a prospective, randomized, controlled clinical study. Clin Oral Investig. 2015;19:1807–14.
54. Karring ES, Stavropoulos A, Ellegaard B, Karring T. Treatment of peri-implantitis by the VectorR system. A pilot study. Clin Oral Implants Res. 2005;16:288–93.
55. Renvert S, Samuelsson E, Lindahl C, Persson GR. Mechanical non-surgical treatment of peri-implantitis: a double-blind randomized longitudinal clinical study. I: clinical results. J Clin Periodontol. 2009;36:604–9.
56. Renvert S, Lessem J, Dahlen G, Renvert H, Lindahl C. Mechanical and repeated antimicrobial therapy using a local drug delivery system in the treatment of peri-implantitis: a randomized clinical trial. J Periodontol. 2008;79:836–44.
57. Renvert S, Lessem J, Dahlen G, Lindahl C, Svensson M. Topical minocycline microspheres versus topical chlorhexidine gel as an adjunct to mechanical debridement of incipient peri-implant infections: a randomized clinical trial. J Clin Periodontol. 2006;33:362–9.

58. Sahm N, Becker J, Santel T, Schwarz F. Non-surgical treatment of peri-implantitis using an air-abrasive device or mechanical debridement and local application of chlorhexidine: a prospective, randomized, controlled clinical study. J Clin Periodontol. 2011;38:872–8.
59. Schär D, Ramseier CA, Eick S, Arweiler NB, Sculean A, Salvi GE. Anti-infective therapy of peri-implantitis with adjunctive local drug delivery or photodynamic therapy: six-month outcomes of a prospective randomized clinical trial. Clin Oral Implants Res. 2013;24:104–10.
60. Petersilka GJ, Tunkel J, Barakos K, Heinecke A, Häberlein I, Flemmig TF. Subgingival plaque removal at interdental sites using a low abrasive air polishing powder. J Periodontol. 2003;74:307–11.
61. Deppe H, Horch HH, Neff A. Conventional versus CO_2 laser-assisted treatment of peri-implant defects with the concomitant use of pure-phase beta-tricalcium phosphate: a 5-year clinical report. Int J Oral Maxillofac Implants. 2007;22:79–86.
62. Schwarz F, Bieling K, Bonsmann M, Latz T, Becker J. Nonsurgical treatment of moderate and advanced periimplantitis lesions: a controlled clinical study. Clin Oral Investig. 2006b;10:279–88.
63. Persson GR, Roos-Jansaker AM, Lindahl C, Renvert S. Microbiologic results after nonsurgical erbium-doped:yttrium, aluminum, and garnet laser or air-abrasive treatment of periimplantitis: a randomized clinical trial. J Periodontol. 2011;82:1267–78.
64. Bassetti M, Schär D, Wicki B, Eick S, Ramseier CA, Arweiler NB, et al. Anti-infective therapy of peri-implantitis with adjunctive local drug delivery or photodynamic therapy: 12-month outcomes of a randomized controlled clinical trial. Clin Oral Implants Res. 2013;25:279–87.
65. Deppe H, Mücke T, Wagenpfeil S, Kesting M, Sculean A. Nonsurgical antimicrobial photodynamic therapy in moderate vs severe peri-implant defects: a clinical pilot study. Quintessence Int. 2013;44:609–18.
66. Mombelli A, Moene R, Decaillet F. Surgical treatments of peri-implantitis. Eur J Oral Implantol. 2012b;5:S61–70.
67. Deppe H, Horch HH, Henke J, Donath K. Peri-implant care of ailing implants with the carbon dioxide laser. Int J Oral Maxillofac Implants. 2001;16(5):659–67.
68. De Waal YC, Raghoebar GM, Meijer HJ, Winkel EG, van Winkelhoff AJ. Implant decontamination with 2% chlorhexidine during surgical periimplantitis treatment: a randomized, double-blind, controlled trial. Clin Oral Implants Res. 2015;26:1015–23.
69. De Waal YC, Raghoebar GM, Huddleston Slater JJ, Meijer HJ, Winkel EG, van Winkelhoff AJ. Implant decontamination during surgical peri-implantitis treatment: a randomized, double-blind, placebo-controlled trial. J Clin Periodontol. 2013;40:186–95.
70. Papadopoulos CA, Vouros I, Menexes G, Konstantinidis A. The utilization of a diode laser in the surgical treatment of peri-implantitis. A randomized clinical trial. Clin Oral Investig. 2015;19:1851–60.
71. Romeo E, Ghisolfi M, Murgolo N, Chiapasco M, Lops D, Vogel G. Therapy of peri-implantitis with resective surgery. A 3-year clinical trial on rough screw-shaped oral implants. Part I: clinical outcome. Clin Oral Implants Res. 2005;16:9–18.
72. Aghazadeh A, Persson GR, Renvert S. A single-centre randomized controlled clinical trial on the adjunct treatment of intra-bony defects with autogenous bone or a xenograft: results after 12 months. J Clin Periodontol. 2012;39:666–73.
73. Roccuzzo M, Bonino F, Bonino L, Dalmasso P. Surgical therapy of peri-implantitis lesions by means of a bovine-derived xenograft: comparative results of a prospective study on two different implant surfaces. Surgical treatment of peri-implantitis. J Clin Periodontol. 2011;38:738–45.
74. Roos-Jansaker AM, Persson GR, Lindahl C, Renvert S. Surgical treatment of peri-implantitis using a bone substitute with or without a resorbable membrane: a 5-year follow-up. J Clin Periodontol. 2014;41:1108–14.
75. Roos-Jansker A-M, Lindahl C, Pesson GR, Renvert S. Long-term stability of surgical bone regenerative procedures of peri-implantitis lesions in a prospective case–control study over 3 years. J Clin Periodontol. 2011;38:590–7.

76. Roos-Jansaker AM, Renvert H, Lindahl C, Renvert S. Surgical treatment of peri-implantitis using a bone substitute with or without a resorbable membrane: a prospective cohort study. J Clin Periodontol. 2007;34:625–32.
77. Schwarz F, Hegewald A, John G, Sahm N, Becker J. Four-year follow-up of combined surgical therapy of advanced peri-implantitis evaluating two methods of surface decontamination. J Clin Periodontol. 2013;40:962–7.
78. Schwarz F, Sahm N, Iglhaut G, Becker J. Impact of the method of surface debridement and decontamination on the clinical outcome following combined surgical therapy of peri-implantitis: a randomized controlled clinical study. J Clin Periodontol. 2011;38:276–84.
79. Schwarz F, Sahm N, Schwarz K, Becker J. Impact of defect configuration on the clinical outcome following surgical regenerative therapy of peri-implantitis. J Clin Periodontol. 2010;37:449–55.
80. Schwarz F, Sahm N, Bieling K, Becker J. Surgical regenerative treatment of peri-implantitis lesions using a nanocrystalline hydroxyapatite or a natural bone mineral in combination with a collagen membrane: a four-year clinical follow-up report. J Clin Periodontol. 2009;36:807–14.
81. Schwarz F, Sculean A, Bieling K, Ferrari D, Rothamel D, Becker J. Two-year clinical results following treatment of peri-implantitis lesions using a nanocrystalline hydroxyapatite or a natural bone mineral in combination with a collagen membrane. J Clin Periodontol. 2008;35:80–7.
82. Wohlfahrt JC, Lyngstadaas SP, Ronold HJ, Saxegaard E, Ellingsen JE, Karlsson S, Aass AM. Porous titanium granules in the surgical treatment of peri-implant osseous defects: a randomized clinical trial. Int J Oral Maxillofac Implants. 2012;27:401–10.
83. Schwarz F, John G, Mainusch S, Sahm N, Becker J. Combined surgical therapy of peri-implantitis evaluating two methods of surface debridement and decontamination. A two-year clinical follow up report. J Clin Periodontol. 2012;39:789–97.
84. Romeo E, Lops D, Chiapasco M, Ghisolfi M, Vogel G. Therapy of peri-implantitis with resective surgery. A 3-year clinical trial on rough screw-shaped oral implants. Part II: radiographic outcome. Clin Oral Implants Res. 2007;18:179–87.
85. Wohlfahrt JC, Aass AM, Granfeldt F, Lyngstadaas SP, Reseland JE. Sulcus fluid bone marker levels and the outcome of surgical treatment of peri-implantitis. J Clin Periodontol. 2014;41:424–31.
86. Khoury F. Surgical therapy of peri-implant disease: a 3-year follow-up study of cases treated with 3 different techniques of bone regeneration. J Periodontol. 2001;72(11):1498–508.
87. Sculean A, Chappuis V, Cosgarea R. Coverage of mucosal recessions at dental implants. Periodontol 2000. 2017;73:134–40.
88. Flanagan D. Implant placement in failed endodontic sites: a review. J Oral Implantol. 2016;42:224–30.
89. Sarmast ND, Wang HH, Soldatos NK, Angelov N, Dorn S, Yukna R, Iacono VJ. A novel treatment decision tree and literature review of retrograde peri-implantitis. J Periodontol. 2016;87:1458–67.
90. Ramanauskaite A, Juodzbalys G, Tözüm TF. Apical/retrograde periimplantitis/implant periapical lesion: etiology, risk factors, and treatment options: a systematic review. Implant Dent. 2016;25:684–97.
91. Salvi GE, Ramseier CA. Efficacy of patient-administered mechanical and/or chemical plaque control protocols in the management of peri-implant mucositis. A systematic review. J Clin Periodontol. 2015;42(Suppl 16):S187–201.
92. Schwarz F, Sahm N, Becker J. Combined surgical therapy of advanced peri-implantitis lesions with concomitant soft tissue volume augmentation. A case series. Clin Oral Implants Res. 2014;25:132–6.

Laser in Oral Implantology

9

Herbert Deppe

9.1 Introduction

It was in 1959 that the first laser was developed by the physicist T.H. Maiman at the Hughes Research Laboratory in Malibu, California [1]. He used a flashlamp-pumped ruby crystal, which produced red light with a wavelength of 694 nm. Almost 30 years later, the first laser for dental applications was designed in 1989 by William and Terry Myers [2], who had modified an ophthalmic laser to dental laser. Within in the last two decades, several laser wavelengths were developed and gained popularity in different fields of dentistry.

This article is a comprehensive review of recent laser applications in implant dentistry, providing information for dentists and oral and maxillofacial surgeons. Therefore, the authors focus on some basic physical information on laser technology, on pre-implantological indications, on osteotomy and implant cavity preparation, and on second-stage laser surgery and peri-implant care of ailing implants including photodynamic therapy. Finally, important safety warnings address the clinician who wants to become familiar with laser technique.

9.2 Laser Basics

For the use of laser in dentistry, it is necessary to understand the fundamental principles of laser light. The word "laser" is an acronym for "light amplification by stimulated emission of radiation." The principle of stimulated light emission was described by

H. Deppe (✉)
Department of Oral, Maxillofacial and Plastic Surgery, Technische Universität München, Munich, Germany
e-mail: herbert.deppe@tum.de

A. S. Budihardja, T. Mücke (eds.), *Bone Management in Dental Implantology*,
https://doi.org/10.1007/978-3-319-78951-4_9

Albert Einstein [3] in 1917. Atoms in a conventional light source, such as a lightbulb, for example, emit light spontaneously. In contrast, laser light is emitted by stimulated emission. In the unexcited state, electrons orbit the nucleus at their lowest energy level or ground state. However, absorption of energy causes the electrons to become excited which means that electrons move to a higher energy level. If such electrons are surrounded by a suitable stationary electromagnetic wave in a resonant chamber between two mirrors, stimulated emission of radiation may occur. This term describes the process by which an incoming photon of a specific frequency can interact with an excited atomic electron (or other excited molecular states), causing it to drop to a lower energy level. In other words, this photon had caused stimulated emission of radiation. During this process, energy is released from the atom because the photon dropped to a lower energy level and the incoming photon is released simultaneously. Accordingly, radiation was both stimulated and amplified. As more and more atoms become excited and then return to ground state within the resonant chamber, more and more photons (i.e., electromagnetic radiation) are produced. In consequence, lasers are devices that emit a single, coherent wavelength of electromagnetic radiation and consist of an energy source, a resonant chamber which generates and maintains the stationary wave and an active medium (Fig. 9.1). As case apart, diode lasers are electrically pumped devices in whom the active laser medium is formed by a p-n junction of a semiconductor diode [4].

The radiation that is produced has unique properties including monochromacy, coherence, and collimation. Monochromacy means that all photons in a laser beam are of the same wavelength. Coherence refers to the synchronization of the laser beam in time and space which means that photons of the beam are in-phase (or coherent). Collimation indicates that the elements of the laser beam are nearly parallel. Due to the little divergence, laser beams can be focused to a small area. This property differs from conventional light which diverges substantially. Because of collimation, the energy emitted from a laser source can be captured and delivered through flexible optical fibers. For more detailed information, specific literature is recommended [5].

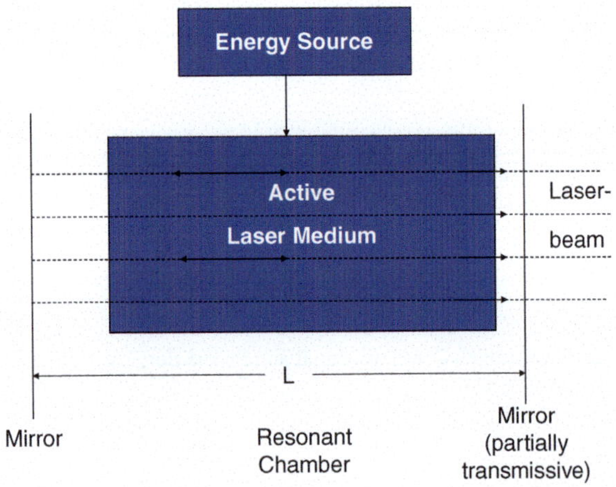

Fig. 9.1 Principle of a lasers device, consisting of an energy source, a resonant chamber, and an active medium

9.3 Laser Effects, Advantages, and Disadvantages

Unlike to other light sources, monochromatic and collimated electromagnetic laser radiation results in unique applications. The effects on the tissue are due to the dissipation of the absorbed energy by conversion to other forms of energy including thermal, mechanical, or chemical energy. Laser therapy of many tissues is based upon the concept of "selective photothermolysis," whereby thermal injury is induced with limited damage to the surrounding structures. Photoablation is caused by mechanical disruption of tissue due to delivery of energy that is sufficient to produce thermal explosions or shock waves within the tissue, thus leading to its disintegration. Photochemical reaction occurs following laser treatment of tissue after injection of a photosensitizer of a specific wavelength.

Whether or not a laser system is suitable for incisions, vaporization or coagulation is determined by the wavelength, energy fluence, optical characteristics of the tissues, and how the laser is operated. In continuous mode, the laser provides a constant and stable energy output. Pulsed laser systems, in contrast, provide alternating bursts of energy followed by short breaks.

According to the literature, advantages of lasers in implant dentistry therapy include less pain, less need for anesthetics (an advantage for medically compromised patients), minimized risk of bacteremia, soft tissue wound healing without scar tissue formation, bleeding control (dependent on the wavelength and power settings), no need for sutures in several indications, use of fewer instruments and materials (economic advantages), and ability to remove both hard and soft tissues, in combination with scalpels (however, the laser is a tool and not a panacea). Disadvantages of using lasers include relatively high cost of the devices, need for additional education (especially in basic physics), every wavelength that has different properties, and need for implementation of safety measures [6].

9.4 Dental Laser Systems

The most common medical lasers emit wavelengths in the infrared part of the spectrum (Fig. 9.2): the neodymium:yttrium-aluminium-garnet laser (Nd-YAG, wavelength $\lambda = 1.064$ µm); the neodymium: yttrium-aluminum-perovskite laser (Nd-YAP, wavelength $\lambda = 1.06$ µm and 1.34 µm); the erbium:yttrium-aluminium-garnet laser (Er-YAG, $\lambda = 2.94$ µm); the erbium, chromium:yttrium-scandium-gallium-garnet laser (Er,Cr-YSGG, $\lambda = 2.78$µm); and the CO_2 laser ($\lambda = 10.6$ and 9.6 µm) (Figs. 9.3, 9.4, and 9.5). Within the visible portion of the electromagnetic spectrum, argon lasers emit a light between 458 and 515 nm, and excimer lasers are located in the ultraviolet part of the spectrum (100–400 nm). Diode lasers emit wavelengths of $\lambda = 810$ and 906 nm.

Lasers within the ultraviolet part of the spectrum are able to ionize tissues, known as photochemical desorption. Lasers of longer wavelengths, especially those within the infrared part of the spectrum (700–10,000 nm), cause significant tissue heating. Most of the surgical lasers are embedded in the latter group and comprised as

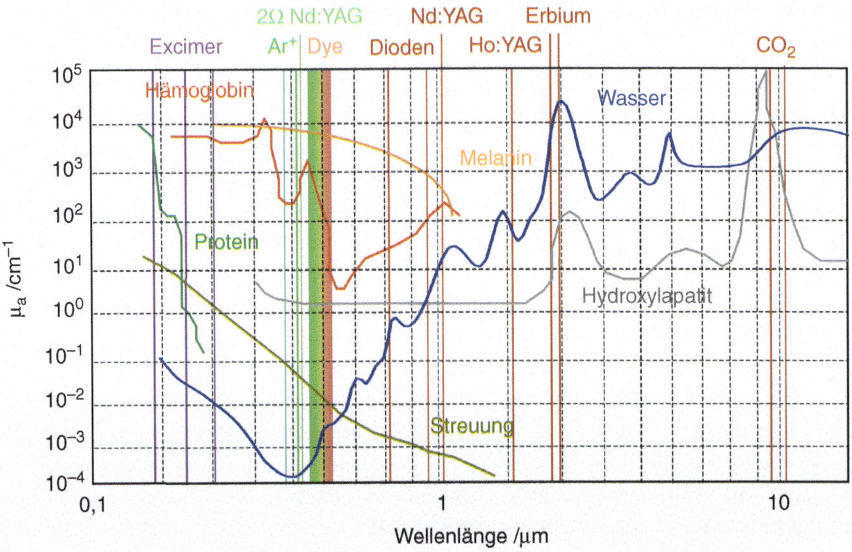

Fig. 9.2 Absorption of medical laser wavelengths (according to Müller G, Hibst R, Ertl Th. (eds): Angewandte Laserzahnheilkunde. Lehr- und Handbuch für Praxis und Klinik. Loseblatt-Ausgabe. Ecomed, Landsberg 2003)

thermal lasers. Light of these lasers is rapidly converted to thermal energy causing denaturation of proteins, decomposition of tissue, microexplosion of cell water and charring.

The lasers primarily used in implantology are semiconductor diode lasers, solid state laser (Nd-YAG, Er-YAG, Er,Cr-YSGG), and gas lasers (CO_2 lasers). Diode lasers, CO_2, and Nd-YAG and Nd-YAP lasers may be used for soft tissue applications due to their excellent coagulation properties; Er-YAG and Er,Cr-YSGG lasers are suitable for the hard tissue applications due to the high absorption from hydroxyapatite. Lasers in implant dentistry may improve hemostasis, result in precise incision margins, minimal damage to the surrounding tissues, and reduced postoperative swelling [7].

A relatively new blue light diode laser system ($\lambda = 445$ nm) for dental soft tissue surgery was recently studied on cellular level. Therefore, an in vitro cell culture model was established to evaluate the effects of the 445 nm diode laser in comparison to an established infrared diode laser (IR). Despite a larger wound area after irradiation with 445 nm, due to its higher temperature development, this laser system showed a faster wound healing in comparison to the IR laser. The blue diode laser system demonstrated an excellent direct thermal coupling to cells and tissues without side effects even by reduced power settings. It was concluded that the blue diode laser seems to be a promising technology for clinical application due to high absorption of blue light without major side effects in adjacent tissues even by reduced power settings [8]. Accordingly, positive first clinical results have been published recently [9].

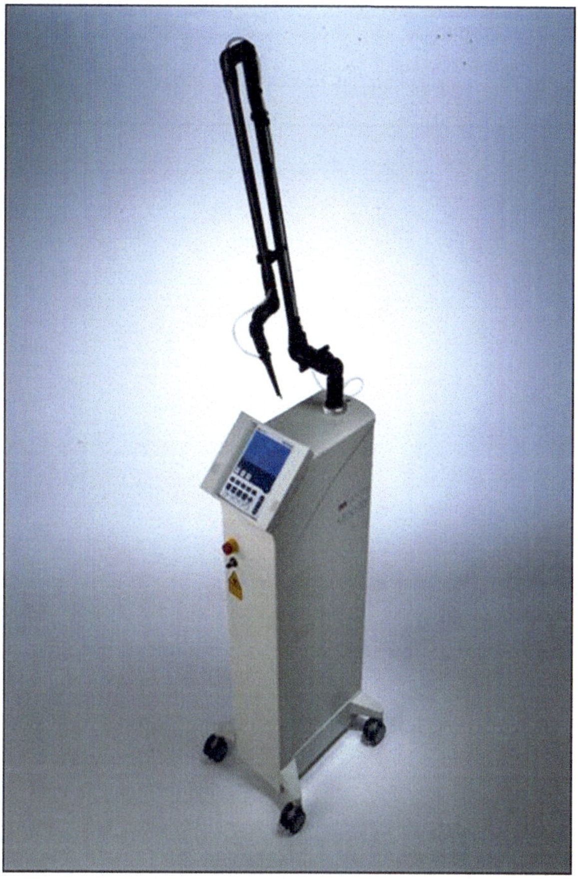

Fig. 9.3 Medical CO_2 laser MCO 25 plus ($\lambda = 10.6\ \mu m$), Martin GmbH & Co. KG, Ludwigstaler Straße 132, D-Tuttlingen

9.5 Laser Indications

9.5.1 Soft Tissue Laser Surgery

Before implant placement, lasers may be used for the removal of granulation tissue and disinfection of the surgical area after extraction, regardless of whether implants or bone grafts are being placed [10]. Moreover, lasers with good absorption of their light such as the CO_2 and Er-YAG lasers are also appropriate for surgical correction of soft tissues such as frenectomies, ablation of lesions, incisional and excisional biopsies, gingivectomies, gingivoplasties, soft tissue tuberosity reductions, coagulation of graft donor sites, and crown lengthening procedures [11].

Hyperplastic tissues can be excised by scalpel, electrosurgery, or laser. However, electrosurgery can result in thermal damage by increasing the temperature over the critical limit of 10°C which can cause implant failure [12]. Therefore, it was pointed out that pain and patient discomfort during and after the surgical procedure is

Fig. 9.4 Medical Er-YAG laser Fidelis Plus ($\lambda = 2.94$ µm), Fotona, Stegne 7, 1210 Ljubljana, Slovenia

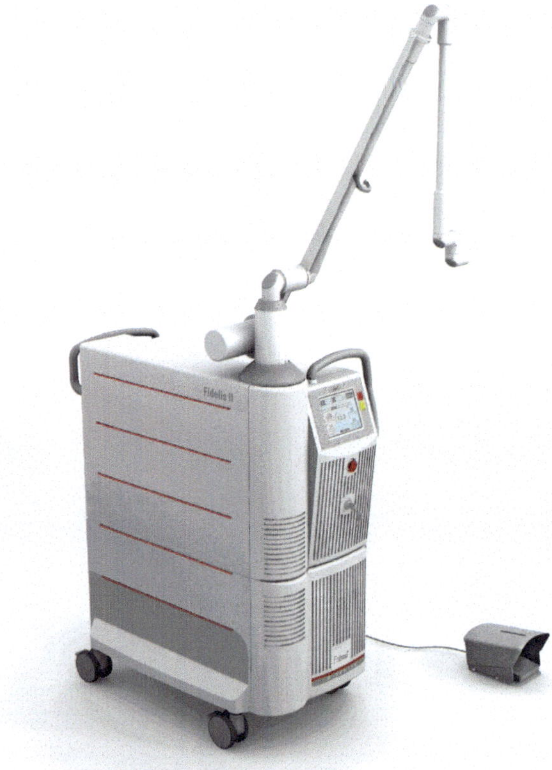

Fig. 9.5 Medical diode laser ($\lambda = 660$ nm) HELBO® Theralite Laser, HELBO Medizintechnik GmbH, A-Wels

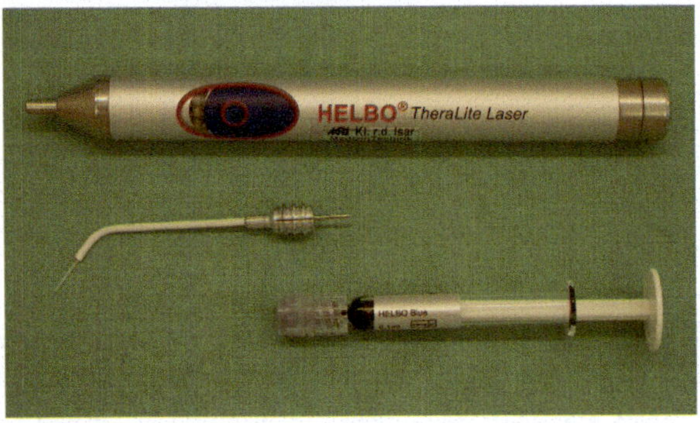

common [13]. In contrast, lasers have advantages compared with other forms of surgical procedures because of enhanced coagulation. Accordingly, especially CO_2 lasers have been used for excision and vaporization of different soft tissue tumors and peri-implant hyperplasias [13].

It was pointed out that some infrared laser systems (i.e., Nd-YAG, diode lasers) must be used with special care because of the higher penetration depth at their wavelength and the possible damage to indirect bone irradiation. Moreover, due to the higher absorption by titanium, such lasers may overheat and damage the implant surface [14].

9.5.2 Preparation of the Implant Bed

For most patients, drills and handpieces are the most inconvenient components in surgical implantology. Therefore, lasers could offer an advantage when performing an osteotomy [14]. Research was focused on most of the medically used laser systems. The major components of bone and dental hard tissues are inorganic structures such as water and hydroxyapatite as well as organic structures (collagen). Several authors described the critical temperature for bone and noted that temperature elevation between 44 and 47 °C may lead to osteonecrosis [15]. The laser light emitted by the CO_2 and the Er-YAG laser is well absorbed by water. The wavelength of the Er-YAG laser, moreover, is well absorbed by water and hydroxyapatite. In addition to a high absorption coefficient for water and for hydroxyapatite with phosphate, carbonate, and hydroxyl groups, the energy emitted by the CO_2 laser at 9.6 μm is also highly absorbed by collagen. Therefore, this wavelength might play an increasingly important role in oral and maxillofacial surgery.

First studies on laser osteotomy were performed in the last century for the CO_2 laser [16, 17] and the Er-YAG laser [18]. Eyrich [15] compared the super-pulsed CO_2 laser at 9.6 μm to the Er-YAG laser and the conventional drill with regard to their respective thermal effects on human bone. Therefore, temperature rise during ablation of human bone was measured. The results of the study suggested that a maximum rise of mean temperature to 1.88 °C (well below the critical range of 7 °C) demonstrated the safety and tissue-preserving capability of the super-pulsed 9.6 μm CO_2 laser. The laser caused an even lower temperature rise than conventional drilling when using this device for osteotomies on larger bone segments compared to small bone slices. Moreover, the laser showed acceptable efficacy with drilling times comparable to a conventional drill.

In another study [15], bony osteotomies were performed in six patients with 60 μs pulses of a pulsed 9.6 μm CO_2 laser (Fig. 9.6). Histologic sections revealed no charring, but a very thin basophilic zone next to the cut surface. Sections of trabecular structures showed a limited coagulation zone of 20–150 μm. The author concluded

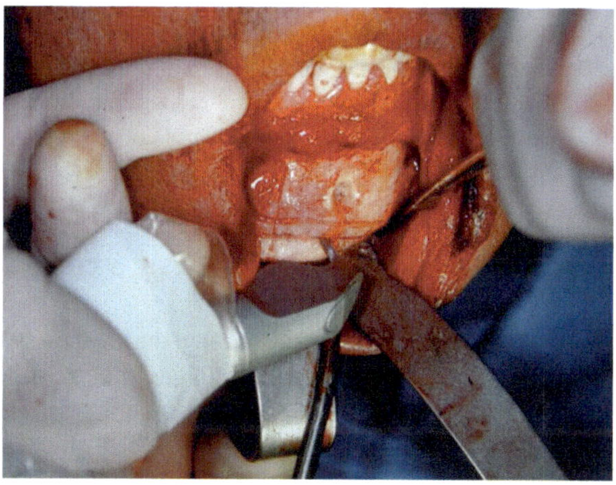

Fig. 9.6 Laser osteotomy with a CO_2 laser device (λ = 9.6 μm) (Source: Eyrich, G.: Med. Habilitation. University of Zürich, Switzerland 2004 [15])

that clinical use of a 9.6 μm CO_2 laser as a cutting tool can be considered to preserve tissue with almost no adverse effects at the light microscopic level.

Similarly, a mechanically Q-switched CO_2 laser, delivering 300 ns pulses at 9.6 μm wavelength, focused down to a spot size of 440 μm on the tissue (i.e., a corresponding energy density of 9 J/cm^2), showed favorable results [19]. Bone samples (blocks from pig femur, rib, or cartilage) were moved through the beam repeatedly until 1–5 mm deep cuts were produced. An air-driven water spray was applied to prevent the tissue dehydration. Subsequent visual and histological examinations revealed no carbonization, melting traces, or fissuring of the tissue. An extremely narrow, 2–6 μm thick thermally altered layer was observed at the cut border in compacta and cartilage. No accumulation of the thermal damage occurred with increasing cut depth. Laser incisions in trabecular tissue were accompanied with a 100–200 μm thick zone of thermal necrosis in bone marrow. It was concluded that such minor thermal side effects make the Q-switched and probably other short-pulsed CO_2 laser systems interesting for hard tissue surgery.

Lee and coworkers [20] inserted 40 implants into two different types of pig rib bone. One group was prepared with conventional drills, and a total of 20 implants were inserted into type I and type II bone. The other group was prepared with an Er,Cr-YSGG laser, and also a total of 20 implants were inserted into type I and type II bone. ISQ, maximum insertion torque, angular momentum, and insertion torque energy values were measured. Results have shown that both in type I and type II bone, the maximum insertion torque, total energy, and total angular momentum values between the drill and laser groups did not differ significantly. Accordingly, it was concluded that the effects of bone bed preparation with Er,Cr-YSGG laser on the relationship between implant stability quotient (ISQ) values and implant insertion variables were comparable to those of drilling.

Stopp and coworkers [21] described a new method for optimized laser preparation of the bone. Thermal damage depends on the laser parameters like pulse energy, pulse frequency, pulse length, and laser beam geometry. To evaluate the correlation between focus position and thermal damage in the bone, an experiment with pig compacta was performed in vitro. The results showed a dependency between the focus distance and the carbonization of the bone cavities. Furthermore, the depth of the produced cavities decreased with the focus distance (Fig. 9.7). Accordingly, the presented new mathematical model of laser ablation of the bone in combination with position measurement of an optical navigation system may help avoiding thermally induced osteonecrosis during implant placement. Unfortunately, this system is not yet available on the market.

9.5.3 Second-Stage Laser Surgery of Submerged Implants

When the implant is completely covered during the osseointegration phase, the procedure is called the "submerged technique" or "two-stage" surgery [22]. There are basically two methods for uncovering the implant, the traditional technique and the laser-assisted technique. Regarding the latter method, the emotional impact seems to be reduced, since laser-assisted surgery is not perceived as a traumatic surgery

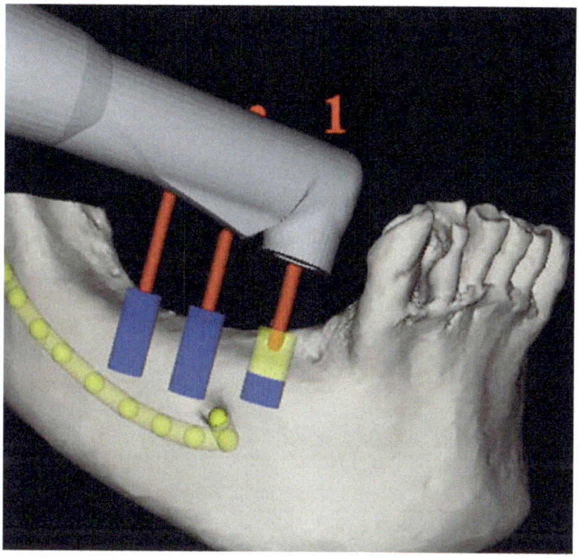

Fig. 9.7 Scheme of combined navigation and implant bed preparation. Bone ablation is calculated by a mathematical model

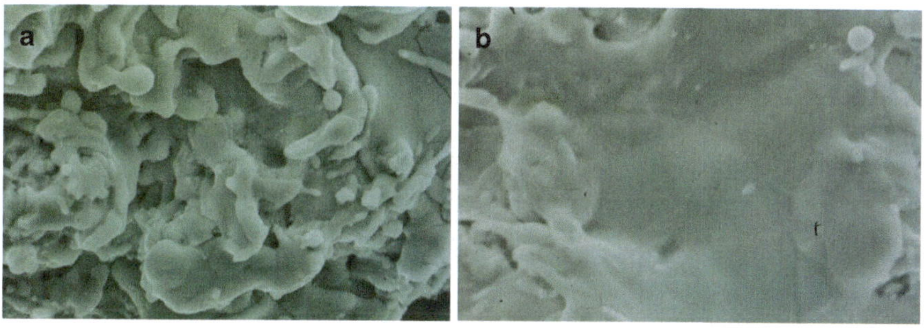

Fig. 9.8 (**a**) Scanning electron microscopy (2000×) of TPS implant following CO_2 laser irradiation (cw, 2.5 W, 10 s). No signs of melting detectable. (**b**) Scanning electron microscopy (2000×) of TPS implant following CO_2 laser irradiation (sp, 2.5 W, 10 s). Large areas following surface melting detectable

[23]. Coagulation properties of infrared laser wavelengths may decrease intraoperative bleeding. The main disadvantages described are the increased thermal stress at the fixture which interferes with the osseointegration and the possible structural changes of the implant surface [24]. Another disadvantage is the necessity to limit the laser-assisted intervention to cases with extensive keratinized gingiva [22].

Fornaini [22] analyzed in an ex vivo model the thermal elevation induced by four different laser wavelengths during implant uncovering: diode (810 nm), Nd-YAG (1064 μm), Er-YAG (2940 nm), and KTP (532 nm, potassium titanyl phosphate) lasers. Four pig jaws were used, and five implants were placed in each anatomical specimen for a total of 20 fixtures. Temperature changes during laser irradiation were measured at bone level, peri-implant tissues, and on the fixture surface with two thermocouples (Fig. 9.8). Surface temperature was also monitored during all procedures with a thermal camera. In conclusion, thermocouples recorded a lower increase in temperature for Er-YAG and KTP laser; Nd-YAG and diode laser produced similar increases characterized by higher values. Similarly, measurements of the thermal camera demonstrated lower increases for the Er-YAG and higher ones for the diode laser. The KTP laser resulted in fastest uncovering of implants, and diode laser was the one that needed most time. This ex vivo study showed that laser utilization with definite parameters is not at risk of dangerous thermal elevation to the tissues and implants. Moreover, after second-stage surgery of submerged implants, impressions can be performed almost immediately due to very little blood existing at the surgical site. Decontamination of the site is an additional advantage of the use of lasers in implant dentistry [14].

9.5.4 Lasers for Treatment of Peri-implantitis

Peri-implantitis is characterized by inflammation in peri-implant tissues and loss of supporting bone [25]. Untreated disease leads to loss of implants [26]. Peri-implantitis lesions are considerably larger and present with more aggressive features than lesions in periodontitis around teeth [27]. At present, there is no evidence regarding the use of anti-infective implant surface treatment to prolong the longevity of infected implants [28, 29].

Many recommendations have been made for treatment of peri-implantitis including studies with different laser wavelengths. A new indication of laser treatment might be the sterilization of exposed implant surfaces in order to rehabilitate ailing implants [24]. However, apparently not all laser systems available in dentistry are of value in this regard. Both Block [30] and Park [31] reported that the potential exists for Nd-YAG laser irradiation ($\lambda = 1064$ nm) to melt the surface and even to remove the surface layer from plasma-coated titanium implants. From this study it was concluded that the use of Nd-YAG lasers in implant-uncovering procedures or peri-implant gingival surgery should be considered inherently unsafe for such procedures [24]. Similarly, adverse effects have been found for the diode laser on high-power settings (>2 W) [14]. In contrast, CO_2 lasers showed less absorption in titanium which reduced the risk of thermal damage to the surrounding tissues [32]. Nevertheless, they provide disinfection and significant bacterial reduction [33–36]. At the wavelength of the alexandrite laser ($\lambda = 377$ nm), structural reactions were seen when fluences of more than 0.8 mJ/cm^2 were applied and at the wavelength of the Er-YAG laser ($\lambda = 2.94$ μm) at a fluence of 7 J/cm^2. In contrast, the authors could not identify an ablation threshold for CO_2 lasers [32].

There are several reports in the literature in which laser decontamination has been recommended including the use of CO_2 laser ($\lambda = 10.6$ μm) [37–39], Er-YAG laser ($\lambda = 2.94$ μm) [18, 22], Er,Cr-YSGG laser ($\lambda = 2.78$ μm) [40, 41], and diode lasers (λ = 810 and 906 nm) [42], both in surgical and nonsurgical interventions.

9.5.4.1 Laser-Assisted Nonsurgical Therapy of Peri-implantitis

Nonsurgical therapy for peri-implant diseases has traditionally been considered effective for mucositis. However, results for peri-implantitis lesions were found not to be effective [43, 44]. According to Schwarz et al. [45], this statement was recently supported by additional randomized controlled clinical studies aimed at investigating different approaches for closed debridement and decontamination of peri-implantitis, such as mechanical debridement and antiseptic therapy with chlorhexidine digluconate, an erbium-doped: yttrium, aluminum and garnet laser, an air abrasive, or an ultrasonic device. In particular, these data have indicated that all treatment procedures resulted in limited clinical [46–48] and almost no microbiological [49, 50] improvements at 6 months. Accordingly, research conducted to date on therapy of peri-implantitis lesions suggests that nonsurgical treatment with an Er-YAG laser can improve peri-implant clinical parameters over a period of at least 6 months. However, it remains unknown whether these effects can be maintained over time. A beneficial clinical effect might be expected over conventional submucosal debridement [51].

Nevertheless, due to the increasing prevalence of both peri-implant mucositis and peri-implantitis [52], there is an urgent need to understand its etiology, leading to the generation of more predictable treatment approached. Accordingly, new laser protocols such as antimicrobial photodynamic therapy were focused within the last years. However, it was shown that a single-stage nonsurgical aPDT was unable to prevent recurrence of clinical signs of peri-implantitis in a 6-month period in severe defects (>5 mm) [42]. Interestingly, most recent literature emphasized exceptional results after nonsurgical decontamination of peri-implantitis lesions [53]. It may be assumed that the key factor was a repeated application of a diode laser (3× for 30 s; settings: 810 nm, 2.5 W, 50 Hz, 10 ms) which was performed at day 0 (i.e., baseline), 7, and 14.

9.5.4.2 Laser-Assisted Surgical Therapy of Peri-implantitis

Renvert and coworkers have pointed out that the presence of a suprastructure, implant design, and implant surface characteristics may limit access to infected sites, and as a result the nonsurgical therapy may be rendered ineffective [44]. Accordingly, open flap debridement with or without the use of adjunctive therapies has been advocated as a treatment for peri-implantitis [54].

However, the use of lasers in the surgical therapy of peri-implantitis is discussed controversely. Schwarz and coworkers [45] followed combined surgical resective and regenerative treatment of advanced peri-implantitis defects comparing an Er-YAG laser device ($\lambda = 2.94$ μm) (ERL) and plastic curets plus cotton pellets plus sterile saline (CPS) for the purpose of surface decontamination. At 24 months, ERL-treated sites failed to reveal significantly higher reductions in mean BOP and CAL values when compared with the CPS group. In both groups, mean CAL values were not significantly different when compared with baseline [55]. However, results from a study performed in beagle dogs have earlier indicated that re-osseointegration occurred following irradiation with an Er-YAG laser [56].

With respect to laser decontamination, Claffey and coworkers reviewed the literature on surgical treatment of peri-implantitis. No single method of surface decontamination (chemical agents, air abrasives, and lasers) was found to be superior [57]. During The Third EAO Consensus Conference 2012, the task of the working group was to update the existing knowledge base regarding the prevalence of peri-implant tissue destruction, the role of occlusal overload, and the outcome of nonsurgical and surgical treatment. It was concluded that adjunctive measures (submucosal air polishing, ER-YAG laser treatment, locally delivered antimicrobials) may result in greater reduction in bleeding on probing and probing depth. However, the outcomes are variable and influenced by factors not yet fully understood [29]. In 2012, Meyle reviewed the literature to summarize current evidence with regard to the decontamination of implant surfaces [58]. This review failed to show that laser decontamination might improve the healing results.

In accordance, Mombelli and coworkers emphasized that the currently available evidence does not allow any firm recommendations for the therapy of peri-implantitis. The following elements of therapy seem beneficial: surgical access by a full-thickness flap, thorough cleaning of the contaminated implant surfaces, systemic administration of an antibiotic, and oral chlorhexidine rinse. The stabilization of the defect with a bone substitute may also be advantageous [59]. Similarly, also the ITI Annual Conference 2013 (Bern, Switzerland) recommended nonsurgical treatment and focused on removal of the biofilm, as first-line therapy. If the disease is not resolved within a 1- to 2-month period, additional therapy is required with use of a surgical access flap [28].

It should be noted that the reviewed literature focused mostly on use of Er-YAG laser decontamination when efficacy of “the laser” was evaluated. However, “the laser” does not exist but a variety of different laser wavelengths, and each wavelength has specific indications [6]. Therefore, more interesting results were seen when reports on other laser wavelengths were taken into account. Application of a diode laser ($\lambda = 810$ nm) resulted in recurrence rates of less than 7% [60]. In further studies, antimicrobial photodynamic therapy with toluidine blue plus diode laser light ($\lambda = 906$ nm) was used in 15 patients with peri-implantitis. Toluidine blue was applied to the implant surface for 60 s, which was then exposed to a diode laser. The results from this study indicated that antimicrobial photodynamic treatment reduced bacterial counts [61]. Haas and coworkers reported on a study in 17 patients in whom the surfaces of 24 plasma flame-sprayed cylindric implants were decontaminated with a combination of toluidine blue (100 μg/mL) and diode laser irradiation at a wavelength of 906 nm. Bone defects were filled with autogenous bone using e-PTFE membranes for retention of the grafting material. Premature membrane exposure occurred in all patients after an average of 3 weeks (±10 days), which required immediate removal of the exposed membrane in one patient. The mean radiographic peri-implant bone gain was 2 ± 1.90 mm after 9.5 months. It was concluded that the short-term results of this study corroborated the efficacy of the applied treatment method in prolonging the service time of dental implants involved with peri-implantitis [62].

Especially, re-osseointegration of formerly contaminated implant surfaces was demonstrated for the first time with use of a CO_2 laser (λ = 10.6 μm) [24].

Accordingly, CO_2 lasers may be regarded at low-power settings as advantageous for peri-implant procedures. They provide disinfection and significant bacterial reduction without causing any alteration to the implant structure [33]. The purpose of a study in a total of 16 patients with 41 ailing implants was to assess the reliability of the CO_2 laser-assisted implant decontamination versus a conventional decontamination procedure [37]. The results of the clinical study demonstrated 4 months after therapy that implants treated with laser decontamination and soft tissue resection showed statistically significant better clinical parameters than conventionally decontaminated implants followed by soft tissue resection. From these results, it was concluded that treatment of peri-implantitis can be optimized using a CO_2 laser-assisted decontamination (Fig. 9.9a–d).

It was also reported by Romanos et al. [38] that CO_2 lasers in conjunction with bone grafting procedures (autogenous bone or bone mineral) demonstrated the advantages listed above. Patients showed reduction in pocket depth around implants with peri-implantitis in conjunction with a significant reduction in bacterial load. Patients also did not experience any adverse reactions such as bleeding or insufficient decontamination during the procedure. Success of the procedure has been documented in clinical cases with advanced peri-implant intraosseous defects which were treated with augmentation using xenografts or autografts after CO_2 laser decontamination [39].

Renvert and coworkers emphasized that despite the heterogeneity of the available studies, it seems that surgical therapy for treating peri-implantitis is a predictable method for controlling the progression of the peri-implant disease and patients receiving this therapy have benefited from it in the short term. The long-term benefit of such therapies is still in question due to the lack of long-term clinical studies [54]. In addition, the authors pointed out that there is marked heterogeneity between case definitions for peri-implantitis in the studies, limiting the generalization of the reported results. Another limiting factor when trying to make comparisons between different treatment modalities is the lack of a standard control intervention. Schwarz [45] concluded that the long-term stability of clinical outcomes obtained following combined surgical therapy of advanced peri-implantitis may be influenced by factors other than the method of surface debridement/decontamination.

Nonsurgical therapy of advanced peri-implantitis cases has, perhaps prematurely, been reported as ineffective and thereby not used as a "gold standard" control. Especially in western societies with an increasing number of compromised patients, nonsurgical modes of therapy might be of value. At present, sensitivity analysis revealed considerable decision uncertainty corresponding with limited evidence about different treatment alternatives for the treatment of peri-implantitis [63]. In a base-case scenario, the treatments that offered best value for money were in descending order: debridement alone, airflow, debridement combined with chlorhexidine chips, and debridement combined with local antibiotics. Er-YAG laser monotherapy, Vector TM System, debridement combined with chlorhexidine, and photodynamic therapy were less cost-effective.

Renvert and coworkers have recently summarized the present status of peri-implantitis treatment [54]. It was outlined that the primary objective is elimination

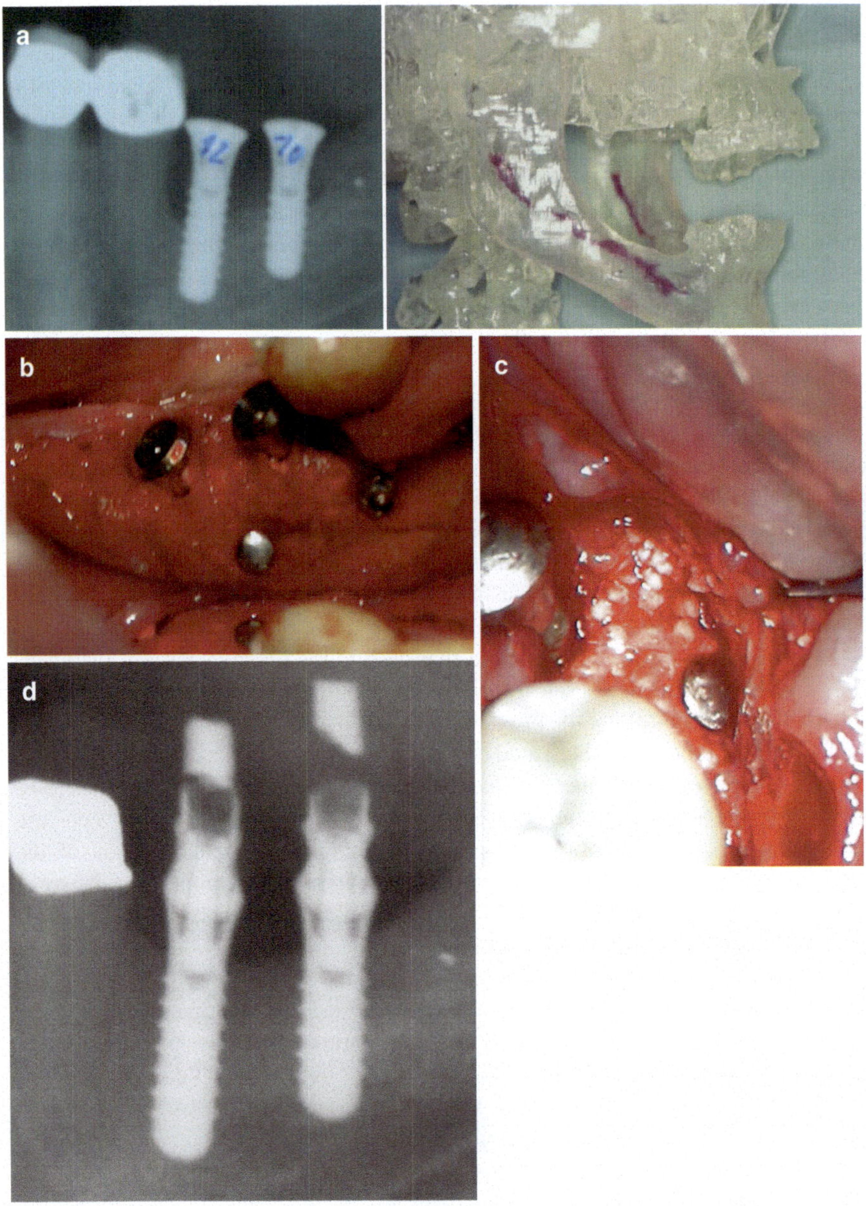

Fig. 9.9 (**a**) Radiography of dental implants in regions 035 and 036 with 50% bone loss due to peri-implantitis. (**b**) CO_2 laser decontamination (λ = 10.6 µm, cw, 2.5 W) and augmentation with use of a resorbable β-TCP, autogenous intraoral bone (ratio: 50:50), and a collagen membrane (Cerasorb®, EpiGuide®, Riemser AG, D-Greifswald). (**c**) Reentry 4 months after therapy: almost complete closure of the defect. (**d**) Radiography 5 years after therapy: stabile re-osseointegration

of the biofilm from the implant surface, and it seems that peri-implant mucositis is reversible when appropriately treated. Nonsurgical therapy is a commonly used treatment. Due to the literature, a combined therapy (mechanical therapy with local antimicrobials as adjuncts) can serve as an alternative to surgical intervention when treating peri-implantitis in cases not suitable for surgery. Surgical therapy is an effective method for treating peri-implantitis, and it is now accepted that following successful decontamination, clinicians can attempt to regenerate the bone that was lost as a result of infection. Finally, a prerequisite for the long-term stability of treatment results obtained is the maintenance of good oral hygiene.

9.5.5 Laser in 3-D Implantology

At present, there is also scientific evidence for the use of lasers in implant planning procedures. Conventionally, preimplantologic diagnosis contains the analysis of adequate 2-D or 3-D x-rays and the analysis of plaster models which were formed with the aid of dental impressions. Based on these plaster models, drill templates are manufactured with drill sleeves. However, in complex cases with considerable resorption of the mandible and flat vestibulum, the conventional dental impression technique can be very difficult. The study casts may therefore not be appropriate for surgery [64–68].

In order to avoid such problems especially in complex cases, stereolithographic models of the jaws can be manufactured from 3-D x-ray data (Fig. 9.10a, b). The method has been described and is well known as "rapid prototyping" [68]. Therefore, based on 3-D data, a blue laser wavelength polymerizes a liquid resin monomer (epoxide, acrylate) and renders layer by layer solid 3-D models [69]. The technique has been used also in orthognathic surgery planning advantageously (Zeilhofer PDZ). The solid model with its hollow structures as the inferior alveolar nerve channel and the maxillary sinus allows an optimal presurgical planning. Thus, the nerves way in the bone and the extension of the sinus can be evaluated before surgery. In cases of sinus lift operations with simultaneous dental implantation, the volume of material needed for augmentation can be determined exactly.

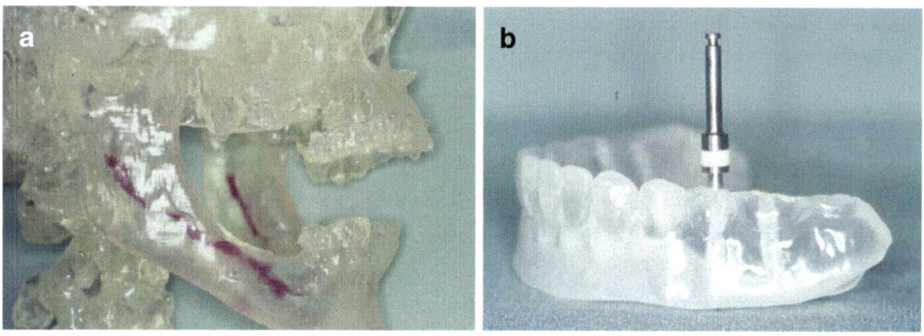

Fig. 9.10 (**a**) Stereolithography model with colored mandibular nerve. (**b**) Drill template, manufactured on the stereolithography model in (**a**)

Furthermore, such stereolithography models can be used preoperatively as optimized articulators for constructing provisoric prosthesis and determining the optimal implant position. It was reported that stereolithography in dental implant planning was carried out in 12 patients with a total of 62 implants which had been inserted based on this method. The authors had seen no damage of the inferior alveolar nerve. Moreover, all implants could be used in the prosthodontic treatment according to the preoperative planning on stereolithography models. Therefore, it was pointed out that the indication for 3-D stereolithography in dental implant planning is complex cases, especially when combined with orthognathic surgery [64]. Moreover, the patient's advising and the visualization of surgical problems can be optimized by using this method. This aspect of stereolithography might become increasingly important in the coming years especially from the juridical point of view.

Based on this technique, 3-D implant planning with use of stereolithographic drill templates has become a widely accepted method [70]. Today, there are three practical methods for applying this technique in a clinical setting: guided surgery by using drill guides which are processed by stereolithographic rapid prototyping [71], computer-milled templates [72], and/or computer navigation systems [73, 74].

Several other laser-based techniques have been used in implant dentistry such as laser-assisted welding, 3-D laser scanning of facial soft tissues, or the so-called augmented reality [68, 75, 76]. For detailed information, appropriate literature is recommended.

9.5.6 Low-Level Laser Therapy and Biostimulation

Many studies have been conducted both on animals and clinically to evaluate the effects of low-level laser therapy (LLLT) [51, 77–81]. For this purpose, the following laser systems were described in medicine with a wide range of dosages (0.2–480 J) and fluencies (6–500 mW/cm^2): infrared GaAlAs and Nd-YAG (continuous) lasers with wavelengths of 820, 830, and 1060 nm, infrared GaAs (pulse) lasers with wavelength 904 nm, and red HeNe (continuous) lasers with wavelength 632 nm.

Dörtbudak et al. [80] have studied the effect of continuous wave diode laser irradiation on osteoblast-derived mesenchymal cells. Three groups of ten cultures each were irradiated three times (days 3, 5, 7) with a pulsed diode soft laser with a wavelength of 690 nm for 60 s. Another three groups of ten cultures each were used as control groups. It was found that all lased cultures demonstrated significantly more fluorescent bone deposits than the non-lased cultures. Hence it was concluded that irradiation with a pulsed diode soft laser has a biostimulating effect on osteoblasts in vitro.

In contrast, André et al. [78] reviewed the literature with regard to the effectiveness of LLLT for infectious pathologies of the oral cavity. Therefore, six articles were selected. Two focused on the effectiveness of LLLT for herpes simplex virus 1 oral symptoms. Two focused on the effectiveness of LLLT for oral lichen planus. One focused on the effectiveness of LLLT for recurrent aphthous stomatitis. The last one focused on the usefulness of LLLT to control stomatitis pain in the hand-foot-and-mouth disease. All the selected studies were assessed with a Sackett's score of IV. It was concluded that no study presented the required quality standards to recommend the treatment of LLLT for the selected indications.

Comparison of the literature on LLLT and biostimulation shows that some effects were described, but widely accepted indications were not yet identified. Due to the heterogeneity and often poor quality of studies [78], definite protocols cannot be stated. At present, LLLT seems to be well comparable to placebo. Accordingly, further studies are required in this field.

9.6 Future Developments

At present, there is a series of interesting indications for lasers in implant dentistry. One of them might be the conservative surgical management of stage I bisphosphonate-related osteonecrosis of the jaw around dental implants with the use of lasers due to the increasing numbers of patients. Bisphosphonate-related osteonecrosis of the jaw (BRONJ) is currently defined as an area of exposed bone in the maxillofacial region that has persisted for more than 8 weeks in a patient on previous or current treatment with a bisphosphonate and without history of radiation therapy to the jaws [82]. The Er-YAG laser can be used for conservative surgery whereby necrotic bone is vaporized, until healthy bone is reached. This wavelength penetrates the hard tissue for 0.1 mm, providing safety guarantees and allowing precision [82]. Recently, Vescovi and coworkers [82] reported on the clinical outcomes of 63 patients treated for BRONJ stage I (according to Ruggiero's staging system). In this study, necrotic bone was resected with surgical drills or evaporated with an erbium laser (Er-YAG laser, wavelength 2940 nm, 250 mJ, 20Hz, fluence 50 J/cm^2 up to 300 mJ, 30 Hz, and fluence of 60 J/cm^2) until the appearance of bleeding bone under sterile saline solution irrigation. It was concluded that that treatment of patients affected by minimal bone exposition (stage I of BRONJ), through conservative surgical strategies, possibly with laser, may result in a high control of the disease in the long term [82] (it may be noted that in 2014, the term BRONJ was replaced by the term MRONJ [83]).

Another promising aspect of future laser applications in implantology may be the laser-assisted modification of implant surfaces [84]. In a study in 24 four rabbits, implants with machined (MS) and Nd-YAG laser-modified surface (LMS) were inserted in the tibia. After 4, 8, and 12 weeks of healing, the removal torque was measured by a torque gauge. The surfaces studied were analyzed according to their topography, chemical composition, and roughness. The average removal torque in each period was 23.28, 24.0, and 33.85 Ncm for MS and 33.0, 39.87, and 54.57 Ncm for LMS, respectively. The difference between the surfaces in all periods of evaluation was statistically significant. Surface characterization showed that a deep and regular topography was provided by the laser conditioning, with a great quantity of oxygen ions when compared to the MS. The surface microtopography analysis showed a statistical difference between the roughness of the LMS ($Ra = 1.38 \pm 0.23$ μm) when compared to that of the MS ($Ra = 0.33 \pm 0.06$ μm). Based on these results, it was concluded that the LMS implants' physical-chemical properties increased bone-implant interaction when compared to the MS implants.

In another study in rabbits, it was evaluated whether laser-induced, site-specific implant surface modifications with micro- and nanoscale topography were able to promote bone formation as compared to machined surfaces. After an early 8-week healing period in rabbit tibia and femur, a 250% increase in removal torque was demonstrated for the partly laser-modified surface. Histologically, significantly more bone was found in direct contact with the laser-modified surface for the implants in the tibia sites, and a similar amount of bone tissue was observed in contact with the implant in the femoral sites. In conclusion, an improved bone-implant interface anchorage was promoted by an increase in micro- and nanoscale implant surface topography and surface oxide induced by topological laser treatment [85].

Moreover, in a recent study, titanium samples were subjected to laser surface modification using an Nd-YAG laser [86]. The glass fiber of the Nd-YAG laser was moved over the samples in a linear motion with 8 W power, 300 mJ/pulse energy, and 50 kHz pulse frequency with 1064 nm wavelength. Following gamma sterilization, the samples were plated with commercially available human calvarial osteoblastic cells with a cell density of 1×10^4 cells/cm^2 per well on a 24-well plate. From the results, it was concluded that Nd-YAG laser surface modification improves the cellular activity, surface roughness, and wettability, thereby increasing the osteogenic potential.

It was the aim of a recent case series study to evaluate clinical and radiographic changes of soft and hard tissues around tapered, platform-switched, laser-microtextured implants 24 months after crown placement [87]. In terms of the full-mouth plaque score and full-mouth bleeding score, tapered, platform-switched, laser-microtextured implants showed statistically significant improvements at 6 months when compared to baseline. Statistically significantly deeper probing depths were found when comparing baseline and at 24 months at mesial, lingual, and distal sites. However, no statistically significant difference was found at the buccal aspects. Radiographic marginal bone loss at 2-year follow-up for tapered, platform-switched, laser-microtextured implants was 0.72 ± 0.16 and 0.67 ± 0.15 mm at the mesial and distal sites, respectively. Accordingly, it was concluded that tapered, platform-switched, laser-microtextured implants maintained marginal bone level (less than 1 mm radiographic bone loss) as well as limited mucosa recession over a 2-year period.

In summary, it may be stated that laser employment seems to have an increasing number of indications in oral implantology. However, further studies are necessary to corroborate this statement.

9.7 Laser Safety

As it was pointed out in Sect. 9.2, profound knowledge of laser physics in association with laser-tissue interactions and training should be a prerequisite before lasers are applied. One ought to be aware that, in contrast to most industrial applications of laser in which the laser beam is enclosed, medical and research use of lasers can expose people unintentionally to laser radiation. Among different adverse health effects of exposure to laser radiation, the risk of retinal injury in the visible and near-infrared regions is of particular concern [88].

The biological effects induced by laser radiation are potentially much higher compared with conventional optical sources due to the special characteristics such as collimation and energy density. Accordingly, most countries have training regulations for personnel who use lasers [88]. It is of utmost importance to establish the position of a laser safety officer (LSO). The LSO is the person who has responsibility for the management of risk and the authority to ensure compliance with all applicable standards and rules. This person should be competent to assess all systems and validate the knowledge and skills of all personnel involved in the laser practice [88].

In particular, Class 3b and Class 4 lasers have the potential to damage the eye through both direct and reflected impact and should never be operated without first assessing the need for proper protective eyewear (Fig. 9.11a, b). To prevent thermal injury, photochemical injury and hemorrhagic injury to the retina, eye protection is essential when operating lasers.

In addition, all persons in the laser team have to be aware that there are another two specific risks: flammability and reflection. Flammability is a potential laser hazard associated with most high-power systems. Therefore, all sources of oxygen should be removed from the laser target site, and flammable gases of any kind should be eliminated in the laser room (endotracheal intubation!). Finally, reflection is a hazard, when a laser beam comes into contact with specular materials, instruments, or surfaces. Specular surfaces may include speculum blades, retractors, non-anodized black instruments, foil masks, or front surface glass lenses. Surface dulling (sandblasting, anodizing, etching) will result in diffusion of the incident laser beam and prevent reflection.

If all persons in the laser team pay attention to the specifics of laser radiation, lasers may be used successfully for the purpose of oral implantology [14].

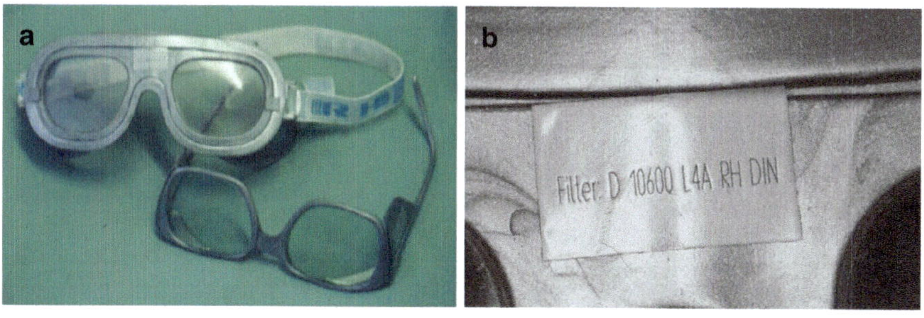

Fig. 9.11 (**a**) Laser goggles for different wavelengths. (**b**) Label providing information on laser protection parameters

References

1. Maiman T. Stimulated optical radiation in ruby. Nature. 1960;187:493–4.
2. Myers TD, Myers ED, Stone RM. First soft tissue study utilizing a pulsed Nd:YAG dental laser. Northwest Dent. 1989;68:14–7.
3. Einstein A. Zur quantentheorie der strahlung. Physiol Z. 1917;18:121–8.
4. Kneubühl K, Sigrist MW. Laser. 5. Auflage. Stuttgart: Teubner; 1999.
5. Berlien H-P, Müller G. Angewandte Lasermedizin. Lehr- und Handbuch für Praxis und Klinik. 19. Erg.-Lfg. – Loseblatt-Ausgabe. Landsberg: Ecomed; 2004.
6. Romanos G. Current concepts in the use of lasers in periodontal and implant dentistry. J Indian Soc Periodontol. 2015;19:490–4.
7. Miserendino LJ, Levy G, Miserendino CA. Laser interaction with biologic tissues. In: Miserendino LJ, Pick RM, editors. Lasers in dentistry. Chicago, IL: Quintessence Publishing; 1995. p. 39–55.
8. Reichelt J, Winter J, Meister J, Frentzen M, Kraus D. A novel blue light laser system for surgical applications in dentistry: evaluation of specific laser-tissue interactions in monolayer cultures. Clin Oral Investig. 2017;21(4):985–94.
9. Skora P, Kraus D, Meister J, Frentzen M. Blue light laser-assisted crown lengthening in restorative dentistry. Laser. 2016;4:6–8.
10. Maden I, Kazak Z. Lasers in oral implantology. Laser. 2013;2:32–6.
11. Pick RM, Colvard MD. Current status of lasers in soft tissue dental surgery. J Periodontol. 1993;64:589–602.
12. Wilcox CW, Wilwerding TM, Watson P, Morris JT. Use of electrosurgery and lasers in the presence of dental implants. Int J Oral Maxillofac Implants. 2001;16:578–82.
13. Romanos GE. Treatment of periimplant lesions using different laser systems. J Oral Laser Appl. 2002;2:75–81.
14. Romanos GE, Gupta B, Yunker M, Romanos Begic E, Malmstrom H. Lasers use in dental implantology. Implant Dent. 2013;22:282–8.
15. Eyrich G. Hard-tissue drilling and cutting with a 9.6 mm CO_2 laser. Zürich: Medizinische Habilitationsschrift; 2004. p. 1–118.
16. Horch HH, McCord RC, Keiditsch E. Histological and long term results following laser osteotomy. In: Kaplan I, editor. Laser surgery II. Jerusalem: Jerusalem Acad Press; 1978. p. 319.
17. Horch HH, Deppe H. Laseranwendungen im Mund-Kiefer-Gesichtsbereich. In: Horch HH, editor. Mund-Kiefer-Gesichtschirurgie. München: Elsevier; 2007. p. 797–820.
18. Keller U. Die ablative Wirkung des Erbium YAG-Lasers an oralen Hart- und Weichgeweben. Medizinische Habilitationsschrift, Universität Ulm: Ulm; 1989.
19. Ivanenko MM, Fahimi-Weber S, Mitra T, Wierich W, Hering P. Bone tissue ablation with sub-microS pulses of a Q-switch CO_2 laser: histological examination of thermal side effects. Lasers Med Sci. 2002;17:258–64.
20. Lee SY, Piao C, Heo SJ, Koak JY, Lee JH, Kim TH, Kim MJ, Kwon HB, Kim SK. A comparison of bone bed preparation with laser and conventional drill on the relationship between implant stability quotient (ISQ) values and implant insertion variables. J Adv Prosthodont. 2010;2:148–53.
21. Stopp S, Svejdar D, Deppe H, Lueth TC. A new method for optimized laser treatment by laser focus navigation and distance visualization. Conf Proc IEEE Eng Med Biol Soc. 2007;2007:1738–41.
22. Fornaini C, Merigo E, Vescovi P, Bonanini M, Antonietti W, Leoci L, Lagori G, Meleti M. Different laser wavelengths comparison in the second-stage implant surgery: an ex vivo study. Lasers Med Sci. 2015;30:1631–9.
23. Bornstein E. Combining multiple technologies to perform minimally invasive laser-assisted dental implant surgery. Dent Today. 2003;22:52–5.
24. Deppe H, Horch HH, Henke J, Donath K. Peri-implant care of ailing implants with the carbon dioxide laser. Int J Oral Maxillofac Implants. 2001;16:659–67.

25. Lang NP, Berglundh T, Working Group 4 of Seventh European Workshop on Periodontology. Periimplant diseases: where are we now? Consensus of the Seventh European Workshop on Periodontology. J Clin Periodontol. 2011;38(Suppl 11):178–81.
26. Derks J, Schaller D, Håkansson J, Wennström JL, Tomasi C, Berglundh T. Effectiveness of implant therapy analyzed in a Swedish population: prevalence of peri-implantitis. J Dent Res. 2016;95:43–9.
27. Carcuac O, Berglundh T. Composition of human peri-implantitis and periodontitis lesions. J Dent Res. 2014;93:1083–8.
28. Heitz-Mayfield LJ, Needleman I, Salvi GE, Pjetursson BE. Consensus statements and clinical recommendations for prevention and management of biologic and technical implant complications. Int J Oral Maxillofac Implants. 2014;29(Suppl):325–45.
29. Klinge B, Meyle J. Working group 2: peri-implant tissue destruction. The third EAO consensus conference 2012. Clin Oral Implants Res. 2012;23(Suppl 6):108–10.
30. Block CM, Mayo JA, Evans GH. Effects of the Nd:YAG dental laser on plasma-sprayed and hydroxyapatite-coated titanium dental implants: surface alteration and attempted sterilization. Int J Oral Maxillofac Implants. 1992;7:441–9.
31. Park CY, Kim SG, Kim MD, Eom TG, Yoon JH, Ahn SG. Surface properties of endosseous dental implants after NdYAG and CO2 laser treatment at various energies. J Oral Maxillofac Surg. 2005;63:1522–7.
32. Rechmann P, Sadegh HM, Goldin DS, Hennig T. Zur Oberflächenmorphologie von Implantaten nach Laserbestrahlung. Dtsch Zahnärztl Z. 2000;55:371.
33. Deppe H, Greim H, Brill T, Wagenpfeil S. Titanium deposition after peri-implant care with the CO_2 laser. Int J Oral Maxillofac Implants. 2002;17:707–14.
34. Kato T, Kusakari H, Hoshino E. Bactericidal efficacy of carbon dioxide laser against bacteria-contaminated titanium implant and subsequent cellular adhesion to irradiated area. Lasers Surg Med. 1998;23:299–306.
35. Romanos GE, Purucker P, Bernimoulin JP, Nentwig GH. Bactericidal efficacy of CO_2-laser against bacteria-contaminated sandblasted titanium implants. J Oral Laser Appl. 2002;2:171–4.
36. Zakariasen KL, Dederich DN, Tulip J. Bactericidal action of carbon dioxide laser radiation in experimental dental root canals. Can J Microbiol. 1986;32:942–6.
37. Deppe H, Horch HH, Neff A. Conventional versus CO_2 laser-assisted treatment of peri-implant defects with the concomitant use of pure-phase beta-tricalcium phosphate: a five-year clinical report. Int J Oral Maxillofac Implants. 2007;21:79–86.
38. Romanos GE, Nentwig GH. Regenerative therapy of deep peri-implant infrabony defects after CO_2 laser implant surface decontamination. Int J Periodontics Restorative Dent. 2008;28:245–55.
39. Romanos G, Ko HH, Froum S, Tarnow D. The use of CO_2 laser in the treatment of peri-implantitis. Photomed Laser Surg. 2009;3:381–6.
40. Azzeh MM. Er,Cr:YSGG laser-assisted surgical treatment of peri-implantitis with 1-year reentry and 18-month follow-up. J Periodontol. 2008;79:2000–5.
41. Miller RJ. Treatment of the contaminated implant surface using the Er,Cr:YSGG laser. Implant Dent. 2004;13:165–70.
42. Deppe H, Mücke T, Wagenpfeil S, Kesting M, Sculean A. Nonsurgical antimicrobial photodynamic therapy in moderate vs severe peri-implant defects: a clinical pilot study. Quintessence Int. 2013;44:609–18.
43. Lindhe J, Meyle J. Peri-implant diseases: consensus report of the sixth European workshop on periodontology. J Clin Periodontol. 2008;35(Suppl. 8):282–5.
44. Renvert S, Roos-Jansåker AM, Claffey N. Non-surgical treatment of peri-implant mucositis and peri-implantitis: a literature review. J Clin Periodontol. 2008;35(8 Suppl):305–15.
45. Schwarz F, John G, Mainusch S, Sahm N, Becker J. Combined surgical therapy of peri-implantitis evaluating two methods of surface debridement and decontamination. A two-year clinical follow up report. J Clin Periodontol. 2012;39:789–97.

46. Renvert S, Samuelsson E, Lindahl C, Persson GR. Mechanical non-surgical treatment of peri-implantitis: a double-blind randomized longitudinal clinical study. I: clinical results. J Clin Periodontol. 2009;36:604–9.
47. Renvert S, Lindahl C, Roos Jansaker AM, Persson GR. Treatment of peri-implantitis using an Er:YAG laser or an air-abrasive device: a randomized clinical trial. J Clin Periodontol. 2011;38:65–73.
48. Sahm N, Becker J, Santel T, Schwarz F. Non-surgical treatment of peri-implantitis using an air-abrasive device or mechanical debridement and local application of chlorhexidine: a prospective, randomized, controlled clinical study. J Clin Periodontol. 2011;38:872–8.
49. Persson GR, Samuelsson E, Lindahl C, Renvert S. Mechanical non-surgical treatment of peri-implantitis: a single-blinded randomized longitudinal clinical study. II. Microbiological results. J Clin Periodontol. 2010;37:563–73.
50. Persson GR, Roos-Jansaker AM, Lindahl C, Renvert S. Microbiologic results after non-surgical erbium-doped:yttrium, aluminum, and garnet laser or air-abrasive treatment of peri-implantitis: a randomized clinical trial. J Periodontol. 2011;82:1267–78.
51. Schwarz F, Aoki A, Sculean A, Becker J. The impact of laser application on periodontal and peri-implant wound healing. Periodontol 2000. 2009;51:79–108.
52. Jepsen S, Berglundh T, Genco R, Aass AM, Demirel K, Derks J, Figuero E, Giovannoli JL, Goldstein M, Lambert F, Ortiz-Vigon A, Polyzois I, Salvi GE, Schwarz F, Serino G, Tomasi C, Zitzmann NU. Primary prevention of peri-implantitis: managing periimplant mucositis. J Clin Periodontol. 2015;42(Suppl 16):S152–7.
53. Mettraux GR, Sculean A, Bürgin WB, Salvi GE. Two-year clinical outcomes following non-surgical mechanical therapy of peri-implantitis with adjunctive diode laser application. Clin Oral Implants Res. 2016;27:845–9.
54. Renvert S, Polyzois I, Claffey N. Surgical therapy for the control of peri-implantitis. Clin Oral Implants Res. 2012;23(Suppl. 6):84–94.
55. Schwarz F, Hegewald A, John G, Sahm N, Becker J. Four-year follow-up of combined surgical therapy of advanced peri-implantitis evaluating two methods of surface decontamination. J Clin Periodontol. 2013;40:962–7.
56. Schwarz F, Jepsen S, Herten M, Sager M, Rothamel D, Becker J. Influence of different treatment approaches on nunsubmerged and submerged healing of ligature induced peri-implant lesions. An experimental study in dogs. J Clin Periodontol. 2006;33:584–95.
57. Claffey N, Clarke E, Polyzois I, Renvert S. Surgical treatment of peri-implantitis. J Clin Periodontol. 2008;35(Suppl. 8):316–32.
58. Meyle J. Mechanical, chemical and laser treatments of the implant surface in the presence of marginal bone loss around implants. Eur J Oral Implantol. 2012;5(Suppl):S71–81.
59. Mombelli A, Moene R, Decaillet F. Surgical treatments of peri-implantitis. Eur J Oral Implantol. 2012;5:S61–70.
60. Bach G, Neckel C, Kekeler G. Conventional versus laser-assisted therapy of periimplantitis: a five-year comparative study. Implant Dent. 2000;9(3):247–51.
61. Dörtbudak O, Haas R, Bernhart T, Mailath-Pokorny G. Lethal photosensitization for decontamination of implant surfaces in the treatment of peri-implantitis. Clin Oral Implants Res. 2001;12:104–8.
62. Haas R, Baron M, Dörtbudak O, Watzek G. Lethal photosenzitation, autogenous bone, and e-PTFE membrane for the treatment of peri-implantitis: preliminary results. Int J Oral Maxillofac Implants. 2000;15:374.
63. Listl S, Fruhauf N, Dannewitz B, Weis C, Tu YK, Chang HJ, Faggion CM Jr. Costeffectiveness of non-surgical peri-implantitis treatments. J Clin Periodontol. 2015;42:470–7.
64. Deppe H, Zeilhofer HF, Sader R, Horch HH. Use of 3 D CT stereolithography in dental implantology. In: Lemke I, Jaffe V, editors. Computer assisted radiology. Berlin: Springer; 1996. p. 1063.

65. Deppe H, Horch HH, Zeilhofer HF, Sader R. Die 3 D CT Stereolithographie in der dentalen implantologie. Z Zahnärztl Impl. 1997;13:79–82.
66. Deppe H, Horch HH, Zeilhofer HF, Sader R. Die 3 D CT stereolithographie als planungsgrundlage in der dentalen Implantologie. Stomatologie. 1998;95:19–23.
67. Zeilhofer HF, Sader R, Deppe H, Horch HH. Treatment planning of craniofacial deformities with asymmetry using solid models (stereolithography, milling) from 3D CT datas. In: Lemke I, Jaffe V, editors. Computer assisted radiology. Berlin: Springer; 1995. p. 1329.
68. Zeilhofer HF. Innovative dreidimensionale Techniken zur Schädelmodellherstellung und Operationsplanung. In: Horch H-H, editor. Mund-Kiefer-Gesichtschirurgie I. Praxis der Zahnheilkunde, Bd. 10/I. 3. Aufl., S. München: Urban und Schwarzenberg; 1997. p. 33–52.
69. Chen LH, Chen WH. Three-dimensional computer-assisted simulation combining facial skeleton with facial morphology for orthognathic surgery. Int J Adult Orthodon Orthognath Surg. 1999;14:140.
70. Sarment DP, Al-Shammari K, Kazor CE. Stereolithographic surgical templates for placement of dental implants in complex cases. Int J Periodontics Restorative Dent. 2003;23:287–95.
71. Di Giacomo GAP, Cury PR, de Araujo NS, Sendyk WR, Sendyk CL. Clinical application of stereolithographic surgical guides for implant placement: preliminary results. J Periodontol. 2005;76:503–7.
72. Fortin T, Champleboux G, Bianchi S, Buatois H, Coudert JL. Precision of transfer of preoperative planning for oral implants based on cone-beam CT-scan images through a robotic drilling machine. Clin Oral Implants Res. 2002;13:651–6.
73. Dandekeri SS, Sowmya MK, Bhandary S. Stereolithographic surgical template: a review. J Clin Diagn Res. 2013;7:2093–5.
74. Widmann G, Widmann R, Widmann E, Jaschke W, Bale R. Use of a surgical navigation system for CT-guided template production. Int J Oral Maxillofac Implants. 2007;22:72–8.
75. Reidy SJ, Lang BR, Lang BE. Fit of implant frameworks fabricated by different techniques. J Prosthet Dent. 1997;78:596–604.
76. Troitzsch D, Hoffmann J, Dammann F, Bartz D, Reinert S. Registration using three-dimensional laser surface scanning for navigation in oral and craniomaxillofacial surgery. Zentralbl Chir. 2003;128:551–6.
77. Abt E. Biostimulation and photodynamic therapy. In: Miserendino LJ, Pick RM, editors. Lasers in dentistry. London: Quintessence; 1995. p. 247.
78. André CV, Bosc R, Chader H, Lange F, Hermeziu O, Meningaud JP. Low level laser therapy in inflammatory and infectious oral diseases. Rev Stomatol Chir Maxillofac Chir Orale. 2014;115:22–7.
79. Bjordal JM, Couppé C, Chow RT, Tunér J, Ljunggren AE. A systematic review of low level laser therapy with location-specific doses for pain from joint disorders. Aust J Physiother. 2003;49:107–16.
80. Dörtbudak O, Haas R, Mallath-Pokorny G. Biostimulation of bone marrow cells with a diode soft laser. Clin Oral Implants Res. 2000;11:540–5.
81. Zimmermann M. Untersuchung zur therapeutischen Wirksamkeit eines He-Ne-Lasers. Dtsch Z Mund Kiefer Gesichtschir. 1990;14:313.
82. Vescovi P, Merigo E, Meleti M, Manfredi M, Fornaini C, Nammour S, Mergoni G, Sarraj A, Bagan JV. Conservative surgical management of stage I bisphosphonate-related osteonecrosis of the jaw. Int J Dent. 2014;2014:107690.
83. Ruggiero SL. Medication-related osteonecrosis of the jaw. Position paper. Rosemont, IL: AAOMS; 2014.. http://www.aaoms.org
84. Faeda RS, Tavares HS, Sartori R, Guastaldi AC, Marcantonio E Jr. Biological performance of chemical hydroxyapatite coating associated with implant surface modification by laser beam: biomechanical study in rabbit tibias. J Oral Maxillofac Surg. 2009;67(8):1706–15.
85. Brånemark R, Emanuelsson L, Palmquist A, Thomsen P. Bone response to laser-induced micro- and nano-size titanium surface features. Nanomedicine. 2011;7:220–7.

86. Charles PD, Anandapandian PA, Samuel S. Osteogenic potential of laser modified and conditioned titanium zirconium surfaces. J Indian Prosthodont Soc. 2016;16:253–8.
87. Iorio-Siciliano V, Marenzi G, Blasi A, Mignogna J, Cafiero C, Wang HL, Sammartino G. Influence of platform-switched, laser microtextured implant on marginal bone level: a 24-month case series study. Int J Oral Maxillofac Implants. 2016;31:162–6.
88. Smalley PJ. Laser safety: risks, hazards, and control measures. Laser Ther. 2011;20:95–106.

The manufacturer's authorised representative in the EU is Springer Nature Customer Service Centre GmbH, Europaplatz 3, 69115 Heidelberg, Germany. If you have any concerns regarding our products, please contact ProductSafety@springernature.com

Printed and bound by CPI Group (UK) Ltd, Croydon, CR0 4YY
25/09/2026
02222863-0008